YOGA AND
VEGETARIANISM

The Diet of Enlightenment

MANDALA
PUBLISHING

San Rafael, California

Also by Sharon Gannon:

Freedom Is a Psycho-Kinetic Skill
Jivamukti Chant Book
Cats and Dogs Are People Too!
Jivamukti Yoga (with David Life)
The Art of Yoga (with David Life)

MANDALA PUBLISHING
3160 Kerner Blvd., Unit 108
San Rafael, CA 94901
www.mandala.org
800.688.2218

Library of Congress Cataloging-in-Publication Data available.

ISBN-13: 1-978-60109-021-8

This book is printed on recycled paper meeting the most strict requirements to ensure sustainable forests. The recycled fibers are processed in a chlorine-free process (TCF). TCF bleaching is a pollution prevention process that does not create dioxins in our waterways or air.

ROOTS of PEACE   ⊕ REPLANTED PAPER   RECYCLED PAPER

Roots of Peace is an internationally renowned humanitarian organization dedicated to eradicating landmines worldwide and converting war-torn lands into productive farms and wildlife habitats. Together, we will plant 2 million fruit and nut trees in Afghanistan and provide farmers there with the skills and support necessary for sustainable land use.

Printed in the United States by Palace Press International.
www.palacepress.com

PALACE PRESS
INTERNATIONAL

10 9 8 7 6 5 4 3 2 1

The content of this book is provided for informational purposes only and is not intended to diagnose, treat, or cure any conditions without the assistance of a trained practitioner. If you are experiencing a medical condition, seek care from an appropriate licensed professional.

YOGA AND
VEGETARIANISM

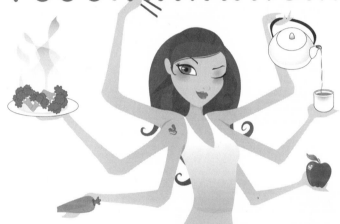

SHARON
GANNON

Foreword by
Ingrid Newkirk

"In *Yoga and Vegetarianism*, Sharon Gannon radiates timeless wisdom and applies ancient truths to contemporary customs. She describes how yoga and a vegan diet can help heal our society's 'disease of disconnection' and remedies a mindset that has allowed cruelty and violence to become normalized on our troubled planet. I hope everybody will read Sharon's book, which describes how our actions affect our world and how we can liberate ourselves through compassion to others."

—GENE BAUR, founder of Farm Sanctuary

"If we are to survive as a species, we need to improve our relationships with animals and nature; this book will show you how."

—DUNCAN WONG, founder of Yogic Arts

"Reading *Yoga and Vegetarianism*...I was enchanted, challenged, and moved. This beautiful book reminds us that loving-kindness is at the heart of yoga."

—KAREN DAWN, author of *Thanking the Monkey: Rethinking the Way We Treat Animals*

"Sharon's mission of ahimsa is so deep and profound; she writes from her heart and soul."

—GURMUKH KAUR KHALSA, director of Golden Bridge Yoga

"Sharon Gannon's commitment to animal rights has been evident in every aspect of her life. She recognizes that the continued murder and slavery of animals affects all levels of consciousness, as well as our health, environment, and global famine, and that it will only be through individual shifts of mindfulness that this suffering can finally end. A modern, compassionate, and well-informed voice for Self-realization and planetary change, she has been unwavering in her quest to educate humankind that our animal brothers and sisters are experiencing a mass level of intolerable abuse that must be addressed if we believe in creating a world that is sustainable, harmonious, and peaceful for all. In her new book, Sharon uses the traditional text of Patanjali's Yoga Sutras to draw our awareness to how our actions affect each other and the world we share. I highly recommend this informative book as an excellent resource to anyone interested in understanding yoga, its principles, and how these ancient teachings can impact ALL beings and species in these contemporary and complicated times."

—SEANE CORN, yoga teacher and co-creator of Off the Mat and Into the World

DEDICATION

To those who want to be free
To those who do not want to be hurt by others
To those who do not want to be lied to—
  who want to be listened to
To those who do not want to live in poverty
To those who are sick but want to get well
To those who want to know the purpose of their lives

This book is dedicated to you, the people of this planet Earth,
  the citizens of this universe, present and future.

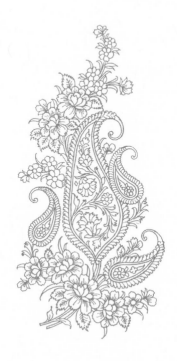

TABLE

OF CONTENTS

Please note: Throughout the book I will use the following conventions in regards to the words *yoga* and *self.* I will spell *Yoga* with a capital "Y" to mean the state of enlightenment and use a small "y" when referring to yoga practices. I will use a capital "S" to refer to the large *Self,* which is eternal and all-inclusive, and a small "s" to refer to the individual ego self.

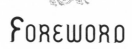

FOREWORD

by Ingrid Newkirk

IN 2008, HIS HOLINESS THE DALAI LAMA, ONE OF THE MOST ENLIGHTENED souls among us, who has lived under threat of attack and death for most of his years, wrote, "Kindness is my religion."

Although His Holiness has experienced more persecution than most, he is certainly not the first great thinker to recognize the overwhelming value of compassion. In the 1800s, the celebrated British writer Henry James proclaimed that there are three things in life that count. The first is to be kind, he wrote. The second is to be kind. And, yes, as you've no doubt guessed, the third is to be kind.

Kindness is the magic word that links, with all-encompassing positivism, every being in the universe to all the others. Through meditation and self-awareness, yogis come to see this interconnectedness that most of humanity only dreams of, yet there are clear and easy steps all "mere mortals" can take to reach this understanding.

Sharon Gannon, the author of this life-guidance book, knows and teaches the vital role of kindness in expanding our spiritual horizons and shaping our personal and collective history. She is one of the kindest people I have ever met, and her deep love for others of all kinds—from mouse to man, from the starving child to the superstar—not only shines through her eyes but also seems to radiate through her very skin. She has that luminescence that comes from inner peace. Her petite frame belies a powerful spirit with the ability—so often lost in the blur of modern life—to empathize with others, *all* others, whether familiars or strangers, and with all the vast animal nations, including our own.

Sharon chose to become a yoga teacher at a time when yoga was viewed by most as a trendy form of physical fitness. She has endured the skepticism of her peers and colleagues in her unapologetic commitment to teaching yoga as a means to enlightenment through compassion for all beings. She has infused her now very popular method of yoga with a strong animal rights and vegan message. Her scholarly understanding of the Sanskrit language and the Yoga Sutras has allowed her to cite yogic scriptural references to support her defense of animals as worthy of our compassion and care. At first her critics told her she was too extreme to bring her own political views and dietary preferences into the classroom. However, she persevered—as all great radical activists have always done—and has made enduring changes in the way that many yoga practitioners, as well as ordinary people, view animals and themselves. She knows and teaches that true spiritual development can only happen through actively extending kindness to all beings.

Sharon learned from her animal friends and protectors when she was just a tot. Humanity is still learning but is often only entertained—rather than enlightened—by the newspaper accounts of studies showing that all living beings are marvelously inspiring and can teach us much about how to live, how to react, and how to cope, if we open our eyes.

It is indisputable that all other animals (for we are but one) share our capacity for love, grief, joy, and pain. Once upon a time, we ruled the Earth with an iron fist, taking whatever we desired from anyone and everyone powerless to defend themselves, including people of other colors and abilities, and it was acceptable to treat animals as inanimate objects. Today, unless we have hardened our hearts and closed our minds to reason, we appreciate them as sentient forms of diverse life, as the "spirits" that they are. We see that we are surrounded by "others" whose lives are interwoven with ours, and we realize that whether they live at the bottom of our garden or are flying over our heads, animals treasure their freedom as much and as passionately as we do ours.

As Sharon makes clear, animals are no threat to us; rather they are our neighbors and allies. Accepting them helps us grow closer to the oneness of life. As philosopher Henry Beston wrote: "We need another and a wiser and perhaps a more mystical concept of animals.... We patronize them for their incompleteness, for their tragic fate of having taken form so far below ourselves. And therein we err, and greatly err. For the animal shall not be measured by man. In a world older and more complete than ours, they move finished and complete, gifted with extensions of the senses that we have lost or never attained, living by voices we shall never hear. They are not brethren, they are not underlings; they are other nations caught with ourselves in the net of life and time, fellow prisoners of the splendor and travail of the Earth."

Through her personal stories and insight, Sharon draws us into other worlds. She reminds us *who* animals are. Elephants weep for beloved lost relatives, prairie dogs use nouns, crows not only use but make tools, mice giggle, cows give a little jump for joy when they solve a puzzle, and birds seek medicinal clay to treat their wounds. She awakens us to the fact that all beings communicate: rhinoceroses use breath language, dolphins perhaps by sending whole pictures, cows recognize their fellows' almost invisible facial movements, frogs use vibrations to drum messages to one another, a squid can flirt with another squid to his left and fend off a squid to his right by creating a message using different waves and patterns of colors on either side of his body, and birds sing at frequencies and speeds too high and fast for us to hear unless we capture the sounds with sophisticated equipment and slow down the recordings. Sharon helps us see that play, a sophisticated concept, is a delight throughout the animal nations, too: that it is not only wild cats and dogs or domesticated ones who roll about with retracted claws and play-bite for fun and tease one another. She asks us to see that we share with the other animals not only emotions but all manner of traits and abilities once thought to be unique to the physically able white man—then to only humans. For instance: fish tell time, octopuses move their finds about on the walls of their dens until they have decorated to their liking, jays play tricks on one another, deer will risk their own lives to stay with an injured mate, and chickens will turn the heater up in their barn on a cold morning if given the opportunity to do so.

These are only a few among countless examples of animals' interests and feelings. Knowing this, we must find it within ourselves, particularly as we strive to be better people, to cast off all hatred, prejudice, and selfishness and to embrace animals as our fellows. Animals are individuals with families who are traveling through life, as we are, vulnerable and hopeful, like us vested with dreams and the desire to escape suffering. This book opens our eyes and hearts to the beautiful prospect of being a far bigger part of life—not apart from life and finding on Earth the very thing our space programs seek elsewhere: connection with intelligent forms of life.

We go through life having many lessons to learn, and those of us who seek to be better people try hard to mold ourselves into beings we can be pleased about, spiritually successful, able to conquer our base desires and striving to be virtuous. By working to extend our kindness to all, without bias and without asking for anything in return, we realize our own potential as good people.

Ingrid Newkirk is the founder and president of People for the Ethical Treatment of Animals (PETA) and the author of *Making Kind Choices* and *One Can Make a Difference.*

Prologue

YOGA STUDENTS OFTEN ASK ME, "WHAT DOES PRACTICING YOGA HAVE to do with vegetarianism?" I hope to answer that question in this book by exploring Patanjali's Yoga Sutras, a scriptural text thousands of years old that lays out the philosophical underpinnings of yoga.

I became a yoga teacher only because I felt it might provide a platform for me to speak out for animal rights. I was hopeful that I might be able to somehow contribute to the evolution of human consciousness so that we, as a species, could begin to see ourselves as holy—as part of a whole.

Some people call themselves "animal rights activists" yet believe that it is permissible to use animals—and even eat them—provided that they are given a nice life before being killed. I, on the other hand, can see no way in which the exploitation of animals for our own selfish needs is ever permissible. When it comes to these practices, I am an abolitionist.

In Patanjali's ancient scriptures, I found the means to articulate—in a compassionate, joyful, and nonjudgmental way—a logical argument in defense of our fellow earthlings: the other animals with whom we share this phenomenal world. Patanjali's words are not only relevant to our present time but essential for the future of all of us.

In the Yoga Sutras, Patanjali presents an eight-step plan for liberation called Raja yoga. The first step is *yama*, which means restraint. It consists of five ethical guidelines regarding how yogis should treat others, all of which clearly support a vegetarian diet. The first yama Patanjali gives is *ahimsa*, or nonharming. Patanjali implies that if we can become firmly established in ahimsa, others will cease to harm us. Many spiritual leaders have noted that there is so much suffering in the world because there is so much violence. If we can reduce the violence, we can reduce the suffering. Patanjali says future suffering should be avoided, and he prescribes ahimsa as the method—stop perpetuating violence, and it will cease. If we could remain enveloped in this state of peace, we really wouldn't need to do any other yoga practice. But Patanjali recognized how rare it is for a person to be truly established in ahimsa, so he was kind enough to leave us a few more instructions!

Billions of animals are killed every year for human consumption after living confined in horrible conditions on factory farms and enduring untold extremes of suffering. This fact alone is good reason for any yoga practitioner to adopt a vegetarian diet. Meanwhile, from the individual health perspective, a vegetarian diet has been proven to prevent and even reverse heart disease[1] and cancer,[2] two of the leading causes of human death in our world today. The terrible toll that eating meat, fish, and dairy takes on our planet's air, water, soil, and whole ecosystem is another reason for yogis, who have traditionally cultivated a close relationship with nature, to consider vegetarianism. Finally, as yogis, ultimately our goal is enlightenment, which involves realizing the unity and interconnectedness of *all* beings and things—not just human beings. Extending compassion toward animals purifies our karmas, creating an internal state of being conducive to enlightenment.

My own journey to becoming a vegan, animal rights activist yoga teacher began when I was three years old. I lived in Florida with my mother, father, little brother, and friend, Mrs. Goose. My parents referred to Mrs. Goose as my "imaginary friend." I did not know what that meant at the time. In my mind, Mrs. Goose was a goose only a few inches taller than I was. We all lived in a big rented house at the edge of the Everglade Forest.

---

[1] John Robbins, The Food Revolution (Berkeley: Conari Press, 2001) 19.
[2] World Cancer Research Fund and American Institute for Cancer Research, Food, Nutrition, and the Prevention of Cancer (World Cancer Research Fund, 1997) 456-7.

One day as we were returning home from the grocery store, Mrs. Goose and I ran out of the car. We wanted to race each other to the front door. As we ran, we both spotted something colorful lying on the stone porch steps. Mrs. Goose told me to slow down and be very quiet. She waddled closer to take a look, then told me to approach quietly. As I got closer, the shiny black, red, and yellow being who was lying on the steps, bathing in the sun, opened her eyes wide to look at us. I had never seen such a creature. She lifted her head to speak. She spoke in such a low whisper that I had to lean down very near to her face to hear her.

I leaned down, and she was just about to tell me something when I heard my mother screaming behind me. My mother came quickly, pushed Mrs. Goose out of the way, and grabbed me. My dad came running with a crowbar and hit the shiny lady, breaking her back. I heard her scream, and I tried to get free from my mother to run and help her. Mrs. Goose was doing her best by flapping her wings, squawking, and trying to interfere. My dad hit the lady again, this time breaking her body into two pieces. My mother let me go. I ran to see the beautiful shiny creature lying lifeless in the sun, one eye still gleaming open, looking at me. As the wind moved through the cypress trees, I heard her whisper, "Why?"

Without intending to, I had caused the death of a beautiful coral snake, minding her own business, sunning herself. I realized that I had the power to influence the actions of other people, for better or for worse, and I had better be careful.

I went to a Catholic school from first to sixth grade. Every morning, the day began with a catechism lesson. In first grade, we learned the Ten Commandments. The day that we learned *Thou shalt not kill*, I came home from school and was excited to tell my mother that we aren't supposed to kill. She was fixing a dish for dinner she called "peasant stew," which had cut-up hot dogs in it. I knew that hamburgers and hot dogs were animals who were killed so that we could eat them, so I was very excited to tell her the news. She responded: "Don't worry. It's okay that we kill these animals because they are raised for it." I went off by myself to think about this statement.

I felt very confused. I had only recently heard the story of Hansel and Gretel and the witch who fattens them up, intending to pop them in the oven and eat them for dinner. I felt bewildered, angry, and disturbed that my mother did not see the connection. I felt even more disturbed because I wasn't able to communicate to her that there seemed to be something very wrong with what we were doing. I realized that if my mother was going to change her behavior, I had to be able to communicate to her in a way that did not make her angry, and for that to happen, I couldn't be angry myself. I had to find a better way.

Years later, in 1982, while living in Seattle, Washington, as a dancer, poet, musician, and painter, I went to see *The Animals Film*—a British documentary that probed into the relationship between human beings and animals. I went because the soundtrack was by Robert Wyatt, a musician whom I admired. Academy Award-winning actress Julie Christie also narrated the film.

Those two hours and twenty minutes in the movie theater altered my life like no other single incident. The film exposed the cruel, exploitative, and inhumane way that we human beings treat animals. The film explored the use of animals as entertainment (from stuffed toys to pets), as food, as providers of clothing, and as victims of military and "scientific" research. It ended with the Animal Liberation Front (ALF) rescuing animals from a laboratory. The movie caused me to radically rethink art, the purpose of the artist, and what I was doing with my life. If I wasn't contributing to stopping the insanity I saw depicted in this film, what was the value in what I was doing?

I had been an on-again, off-again vegetarian before the film. After viewing it, I became a committed vegetarian and, soon after, a vegan. I was deeply affected and vowed that I would find a way to help stop the suffering of the animals I had seen in the film—but how? I tried to voice my feelings, but my friends accused me of being too emotional. It was like trying to talk to my mother all over again. I knew that what I had seen was a glimpse into reality that not many people had or cared to experience. I could no longer live in a cushioned state of denial. I knew that for the situation to change, a whole society had to change—indeed, a whole culture. But first, could there be a change among my friends and myself? Could I change? I felt incredibly inadequate and inarticulate.

While in this state of intense internal turmoil, I fell down some steep, slippery stairs and fractured my fifth lumbar vertebra. The accident resulted in paralysis of my right leg for a painful and frightening two weeks. I recovered the use of my leg, but would still lose all sensation on occasion when the bone shifted and pinched a nerve. During this time, I moved to New York City. My back was still injured, and I began attending yoga classes as a last-ditch effort to do something non-surgical about the pain. Yoga not only helped my back, but the practice also instigated a reintegration of all parts of my being.

During those first few yoga classes, I had the rare experience of going deeper into the feelings in my body as well as the judgments, assumptions, and opinions in my mind. Was it painful? Extremely so! But, perhaps for the first time in my very physical life, I was actually being physical. I wasn't trying to get out of my body—I was actually going deeper into it with a sense of adventure.

Previously I had objectified my body, considering it to be a tool I needed. After all, I was going to change the world, save the animals, and bring peace on Earth—and I needed a body to accomplish this great work!

I realized through the practice of yoga that ideas were not enough to change the world or to change my own life. Whatever I wanted to see in the world around me had to first become real in my own life, in my own body, down to the molecular level. Change had to start with the way I lived, the way I breathed, and how I spoke. Yoga gave me the means to dehypnotize myself from the cultural conditioning to which I—and everyone—had been subjected. Yoga taught me that the disease of disconnection that causes us to say one thing while meaning another—and to do a completely different third thing—stems from a deep lack of self-confidence. Yoga taught me the unitive power of well-being, which arises through aligning with breath (the animating life force) and allows one to feel part of the community of life rather than feeling at odds with it. Yoga taught me, above all, that life provides us with opportunities to be kind. Kindness leads to compassion, and compassion is essential for enlightenment, which is the goal of yoga.

Through the practice of yoga, I have learned something about the nature and meaning of karma. I have come to realize that how we treat others determines our own reality. This reinforced my belief in the reaction Mrs. Goose and I had shared—it showed me that I was not, in fact, alone in my view that we are powerful beings whose actions have an impact. What this helped me to see and understand is that this impact is not just on "the world" at large, but on everyone around me and, ultimately, on myself. That is what finally motivated me to become a yoga teacher as a way to share the benefits of vegetarianism with others who are interested in the path of enlightenment.

I consider myself an activist—a yoga activist as well as an animal rights activist. What does it mean to be an activist? An activist is someone who actively wants to stimulate a change in the world. We all know that pointing fingers and trying to change others is an endless job. If we can't get to the root of a problem, our efforts will only end in frustration.

Yoga offers an effective form of activism because it teaches us that there really is no "out there" out there. What we see in the world around us is only a reflection of what is inside of us. Our present reality is a projection of our inner reality, and that inner reality arises according to our past karmas. Our past karmas are the result of how we have treated others. How we have treated others in the past determines our present reality.

We create the world we live in. If we want to change what we don't like in the world, we must start by changing what we don't like about ourselves. That is a task we can handle and one that will actually succeed in changing the world.

We are in the midst of a global crisis. Most people (humans, that is) don't realize this. Most people don't realize that *we* are causing the crisis. Many of us who are aware that we are causing this crisis don't know what to do about it. I feel that the popularity of yoga at this time of global crisis is no coincidence. A yogi, by definition, is someone who is striving to live harmoniously with the Earth and, through that good relationship, purify his or her karma so that enlightenment can arise. What is realized in the enlightened state is the oneness of being or the interconnectedness of all beings. Such a shift in consciousness has the potential to save our planet.

Lokah Samastah Sukhino Bhavantu

May all beings everywhere be happy and free, and may the thoughts, words, and actions of my own life contribute in some way to that happiness and to that freedom for all.

Let's look more closely at this invocational mantra:

Lokah: location, realm, all universes existing now
Samastah: all beings sharing that same location
Sukhino: centered in happiness and joy, free from suffering
Bhav: the divine mood or state of unified existence
antu: may it be so, it must be so
(*Antu* used as an ending here transforms this mantra into a powerful pledge.)

This is a prayer each one of us can practice every day. It reminds us that our relationships with all beings and things should be mutually beneficial if we ourselves desire happiness and liberation from suffering. No true or lasting happiness can come from causing unhappiness to others. No true or lasting freedom can come from depriving others of their freedom. If we say we want every being to be happy and free, then we have to question everything that we do—how we live, how we eat, what we buy, how we speak, and even how we think.

Karma means "action." It covers all actions—thought, word, and deed. The law of karma says that for every action there is a reaction. Albert Einstein was reminding us of the law of karma when he pointed out that space is curved. Whatever is thrown out there will eventually, but inevitably, find its way back to its origin. So we should be careful about what we choose to think, say, or do, because we will be revisited by our actions in due time.

This may be a difficult idea for some of us to grasp, as we have been so thoroughly conditioned by our culture of slavery, violence, and denial. We have been told over and over again that we don't have to take responsibility for our actions, and that our individual actions don't matter much to the whole—much less to ourselves. But they do matter; in fact they are probably the most important and defining aspect of how our future world will be shaped. We assure our own future suffering by what we do to animals now. These warnings date back thousands of years to the Yoga Sutras, whose dictates are as relevant today as they were then. We each weave our own tangled web of karma and will most certainly become entangled in it, as our reality is being created from our own actions.

The practices of yoga can guide us toward right action and a lifestyle guided by compassionate concern for the happiness of others. The first step toward understanding the link between how we treat others and our own happiness and liberation is to look at the deeper aspects of what the practice of yoga may be able to reveal to us.

Introduction

What Does Yoga Have to Do
with Vegetarianism?

*The most important part of the yoga practice is
eating a 'vegetarian diet.*
—Sri K. Pattabhi Jois

THE SANSKRIT TERM *YOGA* IS FOUND IN THE VEDAS, THE MOST ANCIENT of the Indian scriptures, prehistoric in origin. The Indian philosopher Patanjali did not invent yoga, but he did write an important manual, the Yoga Sutras, several thousand years ago. The word *yoga* is derived from the Sanskrit *yuj*, which means "to yoke," and describes the yoking of one's individual small self to the cosmic eternal Self, or God. Reaching this blissful state of union with the Divine is called enlightenment, liberation, Self-realization, super-consciousness, or *samadhi*. Jesus referred to this state when he reputedly said, "I and my father are one." In all probability, he didn't use the English word "father." Most likely he used the Aramaic word for the Divine, which is *Alaha*. Alaha means the interconnectedness of all beings and things: the oneness of being. A more apt biblical translation of that New Testament passage might be: "I know myself as one with all that is." Jesus was describing Yogic enlightenment.

When Patanjali states, *"Yogash chitta-vritti-nirodhah,"* in the first chapter of the Yoga Sutras, he is giving us both a definition of Yoga and a directive as to how to attain it. This sutra can be translated as: "When you stop (*nirodhah*) identifying with the divisive nature of your mind (*chitta vritti*), then there is Yoga (*yogah*), which is enlightenment." The union of the separate with the whole implies that enlightenment is actually the underlying ground of being and that otherness is an imposition or distortion of a more unified reality.

If we are interested in Yoga, we might ask ourselves, "What is Yoga interested in?" Yoga has one goal: enlightenment, a state in which the separateness of self and other dissolves in the realization of the oneness of being. What holds us back from that realization is a false perception of reality. Instead of perceiving oneness, we see separateness, disconnection, and otherness. Because the term Yoga refers not only to the goal of enlightenment but also to the practical method for reaching that goal, all of the practices must address the basic issue of "other." Otherness is the main obstacle to enlightenment. Killing or harming others is not the best way to overcome that obstacle. How we perceive and relate to the others in our lives determines whether or not enlightenment arises.

When most people think of yoga, they think of the physical postures taught in yoga classes. This is a yoga practice called *asana*. It is one of the many yoga practices, such as meditation, *pranayama* (breathing exercises), and *yama* (restraint), that can help us realize our true nature. The practice of asana, for example, is the perfection of one's relationship to the Earth. What is a perfect relationship? One that is not one-sided or selfish but mutually beneficial. If we are still eating meat, fish, or dairy products, we might question whether or not our relationship to the animals we are eating is mutually beneficial and, with that answer, decide if our eating choices serve our ultimate goal: the attainment of Yoga.

Compassion brings about the arising of enlightenment. All yoga practices are designed to help one develop compassion and, by means of compassion, dissolve the illusion of otherness. Through practice you begin to realize that everyone else in your life is really coming from inside you. Through compassion you are not only able to acknowledge this but also absorb everyone back into the fullness (or emptiness) of your own being. In Yogic terminology this is referred to as *shunyata*—emptiness (or fullness, if you want to see it that way).

Our experience of everything we see and everyone we meet is colored by our own perceptions. We are actually the most important people in our lives because we determine who the others are and what significance they hold. This is not a subjective occurrence that happens consciously in the moment of perception, but rather a conditioned response developed over time through repeated actions or karmas. These karmas plant the seeds that create our understanding of others, of reality, and of ourselves.

Yoga teaches us that we can have whatever we may want in life if we are willing to provide it for others first. In fact, whatever we are experiencing in our lives is a direct result of how we have treated others in our past. The way we treat others will determine how others treat us. After all, they are only acting as agents of our own karmas. How others treat us will influence how we see ourselves. How we see ourselves will greatly determine who we are, and who we are will be revealed in our actions.

The others in our world can provide us with the opportunities we need to evolve. The world will either keep us in bondage or provide us with the means to liberation. When we give to others that which we want for ourselves—when an action is selfless—it leads to the type of karma that will eventually lead to liberation.

As yogis seeking liberation, we strive to perfect our actions. Every action is preceded by a thought. To perfect an action, we must therefore first perfect our thoughts. What is a perfect thought? A perfect thought is one devoid of selfish motive: free of anger, greed, hate, jealousy, and the like.

If you wish to truly step into transcendental reality and have a lighter impact on the planet, adopting a compassionate vegetarian diet is a good place to start. Not everyone can stand on his or her head every day, but everyone eats. You can practice compassion three times a day when you sit down to eat. This is one of the many reasons that so many yoga practitioners choose to be vegetarians.

Ethical vegetarians eat only plant-based food in order to show compassion toward animals and other humans and to benefit the planet. Some people say they are vegetarian but still eat milk products, eggs, and fish. Ethical vegetarians do not eat dairy products, eggs, and fish because these are not vegetables and eating them causes great harm to other beings and the planet. Vegans are ethical vegetarians who seek to extend their ethics to include not just what they eat but everything they consume: food, clothing, medicine, fuel, and entertainment, to name a few. When I use the term *vegetarianism* in this book, I am referring to ethical vegetarianism or veganism.

The term *veganism* was coined in 1944 by Donald Watson (1910–2005), who founded the Vegan Society in England. Vegans do their best to refrain from exploiting animals for any reason and believe that animals do not exist as slaves to serve human beings. A vegan is a strict vegetarian who abstains from eating or using any products that have been derived from animal sources. The mission statement of People for the Ethical Treatment of Animals (PETA) sums it up this way: Animals are not ours to use for food, clothing, laboratory experimentation, entertainment, or any other exploitative purpose.

Some meat eaters defend their choice by saying that it is natural, because animals eat one another in the wild. When people bring this up as a rationale for eating meat, I remind them that the animals that end up on our plates aren't those who eat one another in the wild. The animals we exploit for food are not the lions, tigers, and bears of the world. We eat the gentle ones—vegan animals who, if given the choice, would never eat the flesh of other animals, although they are forced to do so on today's farms when they are fed "enriched feed" containing rendered animal parts.

Some may say a vegan diet is difficult to follow. What does difficult mean? How difficult is it to suffer and die from heart disease caused by a diet high in saturated fats and cholesterol? Still, many people would choose to go through invasive bypass surgery or have a breast, colon, or rectum removed and take powerful pharmaceutical drugs for the rest of their lives rather than change their diets because they think veganism is drastic and extreme. How difficult is it for the beings who suffer degrading confinement and cruel slaughter, dying for our dining convenience? How difficult is it for all of us to be confronted with the effects of global warming, deforestation, species extinction, water, soil, and air pollution that are a direct result of raising confined animals for food? How difficult is it for us to endure being hurt and abused, being lied to, worrying about money and security, experiencing mental and physical illnesses, and not knowing what is in store for us next?

By following the yamas prescribed in Patanjali's Yoga Sutras, we begin to realize that suffering is inevitable only to those who are unenlightened about the truth, which connects us all. Our own actions bring about the situation we live in. Yoga has the potential to heal the disease that we are all suffering from—the disease of disconnection. War, destruction of the environment, extinction of species, global warming, and even domestic violence—all of these stem from the disease of disconnection. You can only abuse and exploit others if you feel disconnected from them and have no idea about the potency inherent in your own actions. If you feel connected, you know that it's *you*, as well as other living things, who will suffer from the suffering you inflict.

It is wise for the yogi to consider that killing and eating another being perpetuates the wheel of *samsara*—the cycle of birth, life, and death. The yoga practitioner is attempting to be free of samsara and, therefore, would want to step out of the so-called natural cycle of the dog-eat-dog world. Some may argue that human beings have been doing certain activities "forever" and that, therefore, they are normal, natural, and should be allowed to continue. The fact that a belief or behavior is long-held does not make it inherently just, or even right. Consider, for example, the fact that men have been raping women for thousands of years. Does this mean that such behavior is normal and should be allowed to continue? We are fortunate enough to live in an era in which human beings have come to recognize rape as a crime. A yogi investigates *all* long-standing habits and behaviors, even if they have been in place seemingly forever, and asks: "Is this activity necessary now? Does it bring me or the world closer to enlightenment or peace?"

Eating meat is a long-standing habit in our culture. Many Western yoga practitioners argue that they have to eat meat to keep up the strength required for a physically demanding asana practice. Yet Sri K. Pattabhi Jois, the Indian master of the physically demanding style of Ashtanga yoga, has stated clearly that a vegetarian diet is a requirement for the practice of yoga. He was initially very reluctant to teach Western students because they were meat eaters. It was only in the last twenty years or so that he opened his doors wide to Western students. I had assumed the reason was that he felt there would be language difficulties, but when I asked him if that was why he refused Western students for many years, he replied: "No. It was because they weren't vegetarians. If someone is not a vegetarian, they won't be able to learn yoga. They will be too stiff in their body and their mind."

"But, Guruji," I said, "you teach mostly Western students now. What caused you to change?"

"In my country, we are vegetarians because our parents are; we were born that way," he replied. "At first when Westerners came to me, I assumed a lot about them. Most Indian people do. But then some students came to me, and I learned that they were vegetarians, and they weren't born that way. They had decided on their own to become vegetarians. This seemed very unusual, and I felt that it was interesting and significant. And so I began teaching them because I felt they could learn."

The popularity of yoga worldwide has grown tremendously in the midst of a global crisis. This is no coincidence. Yoga holds the promise that could help us transform our ways of relating to animals, the Earth, and one another. Through yoga practice, we purify our past karmas and in turn develop self-confidence. We begin to feel like integrated beings as we start to heal the disease of disconnection that has separated our hearts from our minds and our bodies. Then the illusion that we are separate from the rest of creation begins to dissolve. With that disconnection dissolved, we begin to perceive our connection to the Divine, and the truth of who we really are is revealed.

I am thankful that yoga is being embraced in our Western culture by a growing minority, because we desperately need to stop viewing the Earth and all other beings as ours to exploit. Much of our culture's influence has been negative and quite destructive. It is based on the lie that "the Earth belongs to us." Yoga has always opposed this proprietary worldview and has offered humanity an alternative over the centuries: the means to live harmoniously with the Earth and all beings. If human beings can't find a new way to live *with* this planet, then our own annihilation as well as the planet's is certain. Without planetary harmony, no cosmic harmony can be hoped for. I believe that the teachings and practices of yoga are very important, perhaps even crucial, for the survival of life on Earth. That is why I am passionate about practicing and teaching yoga.

The choice to become yogis and the choices we make about what to eat are karmic, political, and economic decisions that affect our mental and physical health. They have repercussions in our families as well as in our larger communities. It is an indisputable fact that a vegan diet causes less harm to ourselves, to animals, to plants, and to the Earth. To say that what you choose to eat is nobody else's business is to belittle yourself and deny the impact that your actions have upon the lives of others.

The biggest consumer of fresh water is the meat and dairy industry. It is also responsible for most of the water pollution. The livestock industry is the single biggest contributor to global warming, as it creates far more greenhouse gas emissions than all forms of transportation combined![3] There are more cows (most of them hidden from our view) in the United States than there are human beings. By enslaving these animals and abusing them through lifelong torture and degradation, we deprive them of their freedom and happiness. How can we ourselves hope to be free or happy when our own lives are rooted in depriving others of the very thing we say we value most in life—the freedom to pursue happiness? If you want to bring more peace and happiness into your own life, the way to do so is to stop causing violence and unhappiness in the lives of others. Yoga reminds us that all of life is sacred, that all of life is connected, and that what we do to another we eventually do to ourselves. The best way to uplift our own lives is to do all we can to uplift the lives of others.

---

[3] Henning Stanfield, Pierre Gerber, Tom Wassenaar, Vincent Castel, and Mauricio Rosales, Livestock's Long Shadow: Environmental Issues and Options (Food and Agriculture Organization of the United Nations, 2006).

How we behave toward others and our environment reveals—more than anything else—our inner state of mind and the current condition of our personalities. How have we become so estranged from our true Divine nature and from nature herself? Are human beings naturally violent, deceitful, selfish, manipulative, and greedy? Or have we learned and perfected these negative traits over time? Could the practice of yoga not only challenge the basic assumptions expressed by these negative traits but reverse them and, in doing so, allow us to recreate ourselves, our societies, and the world we live in?

In the Yoga Sutras, Patanjali lays out an eight-limbed plan for liberation called Raja yoga. The first limb is called *yama*, which means restraint, and includes five ethical restrictions.

ahimsa satya asteya brahmacharya aparigraha yamah
PYS II.30

1. ahimsa: nonharming
2. satya: truthfulness
3. asteya: nonstealing
4. brahmacharya: continence
5. aparigraha: greedlessness

The yamas describe how an unenlightened person who desires Yoga should restrict his or her behavior toward others. Patanjali says that as long as you still perceive "others" and not one interconnected reality, then (1) don't harm others, (2) don't deceive them, (3) don't steal from them, (4) don't manipulate them sexually, and (5) don't be greedy, selfishly depriving them of sustenance and happiness. Through the practice of yama, Patanjali tells us that we can begin to purify our karmas and remove the obstacles to our enlightenment, which are rooted in our misperception of others.

In this book, we investigate how the yamas relate to vegetarianism, as well as what one can expect as a result of being established in the practice of each of the yamas. This is called *pratishthayam*, which means "to become established in." Patanjali suggests that if we work for the freedom of other beings, we will become free. By becoming established in the practice of the yamas, we can look forward to a peaceful world free of violence (through *ahimsa*), lies (through *satya*), and stealing (through *asteya*); the enjoyment of physical and mental vitality and the end of disease (through *brahmacharya*); and a future free of poverty and bright with opportunities for increased happiness and creativity (through *aparigraha*).

What would we find if we were to investigate the yamas in terms of how we are treating the animals we put on our plates every day? Are we harming them? Are we deceiving them? Are we stealing from them? Are we manipulating them sexually? Are we impoverishing them through our greed? What impact does our treatment of these "other" animals have upon our inner and outer environment?

Don't wait for a better world. Start now to create a world of harmony and peace. It is up to you, and it always has been! You may even find the solution at the end of your fork.

Reduce your chances of reincarnating as a cow: drink soymilk!

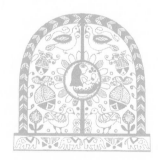

Chapter 1

ASANA

Our Connection to the Earth and All Beings

*We have come into this world to bring peace and happiness
to all beings. To achieve this goal, it is necessary to adopt
peaceful ways of harmless living and noninterference in
the happiness of others.*

—Swami Nirmalananda

*We have been at war with the other creatures of this Earth
ever since the first human hunter set forth with spear into
the primeval forest. Human imperialism has everywhere
enslaved, oppressed, murdered, and mutilated the animal
peoples. All around us lie the slave camps we have built
for our fellow creatures, factory farms and vivisection
laboratories, Dachaus and Buchenwalds for the conquered
species. We slaughter animals for our food, force them to
perform silly tricks for our delection, gun them down and
stick hooks in them in the name of sport. We have torn
up the wild places where once they made their homes.
Speciesism is more deeply entrenched within us than
sexism, and that is deep enough.*

—Ron Lee, founder of the Animal Liberation Front

sthira-sukham asanam PYS II.46
The connection to the Earth should be steady and joyful.

sthira: steady

sukham: joyful

asanam: seat (connection to the Earth)

WHEN MOST PEOPLE THINK OF YOGA, THEY THINK OF THE PHYSICAL postures called *asana*. In fact, Patanjali mentions asana only twice in the Yoga Sutras, but when he does he provides us with a powerful means to purify our relationships with others.

There is a misperception that asana is done in preparation for the "higher" yogic practices, such as meditation. This is not true. In the Yoga Sutras, Patanjali gives asana equal importance to meditation as a practice for reaching awareness of the oneness of all being.

Sthira means "steady," and *sukham* means "joyful and comfortable." In our contemporary times, asana is usually translated as "pose" or "posture." The original meaning of the Sanskrit word is "seat." (The English word *ass* is derived from asana.) Patanjali is addressing those who seek enlightenment. He tells them that, in order to achieve enlightenment, their connection (or relationship) to the Earth—which refers to all beings and things—must be both steady and joyful. Currently, our connection to the Earth is dangerously out of balance, and asana practice can provide much-needed insight into how to improve it.

Asana practice is beneficial on many levels. It has been shown to help restore flexibility and strength, to be therapeutic for injuries, and to balance hormonal secretions, supporting youthfulness. For one who desires enlightenment, asana practice is especially valuable, because it provides an opportunity to purify one's karmas. Because our bodies are storehouses for all of our past karmas, and our physical bodies are made from the food that we eat, imbalances show up as tightness, uptightness, discomfort, and even disease. Through the deeply therapeutic practice of asana, we begin to purify our karmas, thereby healing our past relationships with others and reestablishing a steady and joyful connection with the Earth, which means all of life.

With *sthira-sukham asanam*, Patanjali is proposing a radical idea, which, if realized and put into practice, could stop the war that human beings have been waging against animals and Mother Nature for the past ten thousand years. With the conclusion of that war, we could begin to build a new world and a harmonious and sustainable way of living based on joy and mutual benefit.

Is there a contradiction between spirituality and veganism, environmentalism, or animal rights activism? The latter three are associated with politics, and many yogis have been cautioned not to mix spirituality with politics. But let's look deeper into what the word *politic* really means. *Politic* means "body." The word can also mean the greater body, implying the extended body or community. Being political means to care about the politic—the community of others we live with. The term *dharma* literally means "to hold together," which is what a body does. In this sense, being politically active has a dharmic connotation. To choose to be aware of how one's actions may affect others is to become politically active. To care about other beings and act on their behalf is therefore very much in line with the teachings of yoga.

If we, as a species, are ever going to find a way to live peacefully—which implies fearlessly—then we must look to our relationship with creation itself to see where the obstacles to peace arise. The practice of asana allows us to investigate our physiology and psychology. If we have been eating meat and dairy products, we have bodies that are not only filled with toxins hazardous to our health (in the form of pesticides, herbicides, antibiotics, and other pharmaceutical drugs) but also composed of the karmic results of violence, cruelty, fear, terror, and despair. Through asana practice, we begin to notice how our diet may be contributing to tightness and constriction in our bodies and minds and an uneasy feeling of imbalance with ourselves and others.

We may also notice, as we go deeper into our asana practice, that the prevalent disease in our culture is low self-esteem. Perhaps we feel bad about ourselves if we can't execute a yoga posture perfectly. As we watch our thoughts spin into a downward spiral, we may begin to realize that our culture has done an excellent job of making us all feel fearful and quite inadequate. This lack of self-confidence may cause us to think that what we do as an individual doesn't matter much to the whole and that our actions are insignificant. If we feel this way, we may not believe that we are responsible for our own lives and that we have a profound effect upon the lives of others and the world around us. We may even feel unworthy of spiritual attainment and think that enlightenment is only reserved for people like Ramakrishna, Buddha, or Mother Teresa. The practice of yoga has the power to shatter and dissolve these misconceptions, but it might take a lot of transformational work to accomplish that.

Ours is not a meditative, self-reflecting culture. We are a distracted, gotta-get-up-and-do-something culture, always seeking stimulation from the outside. For a meat eater to be calm enough to come to a yoga mat or meditation cushion and surrender to deep contemplation can be quite difficult, perhaps because it will be hard to bear the truth of what might be found inside: the shadow that has been denied. From its inception, our culture has participated in the brutal reality of the enslavement and eating of animals. If we eat meat, we carry in our bodies the karmic repercussions of the pain we have inflicted upon these animals we are consuming. Even if we are vegetarians and don't eat animals we still live in an atmosphere where this is happening, and on some level we feel the suffering.

Through the benefits that arise from practicing yoga, and not just from reading or hearing about it, we may discover that cultivating kindness improves our sense of well-being, our peace of mind, and our physical health. On the other hand, violence and selfish habits lead ultimately to physical, mental, spiritual, and environmental breakdown.

"Most people's relationship to animals occurs three times a day when they sit down to eat them—that's a terrible way to define a relationship!" says activist Ingrid Newkirk. Contrary to popular belief, the animal nations do not belong to us, and we will ultimately not benefit by exploiting them for our short-sighted gain. The yogi strives to live in harmony with Mother Nature and, through her blessings, attain enlightenment—the knowledge of the absolute reality. This is the underlying reason that eating a vegan diet, which minimizes one's exploitation of animals and the environment, is of vital importance. Eating a vegetarian diet can contribute more to saving ourselves and the planet than any other single effort.

Our meat-eating culture not only affects the animals that are tortured and killed but also causes tremendous worldwide environmental devastation—which scientists loudly proclaim will have catastrophic effects on the planet.

Some facts:

1. Global warming: According to the United Nations, raising animals for food creates more greenhouse gas emissions than all the transportation (cars, trucks, trains, buses, planes, ships, etc.) in the world.[4] This is the *real* "inconvenient truth."

---

[4] Stanfield, et al, <u>Livestock's Long Shadow</u>.

2. Water pollution: In the United States, raising animals for food causes more water pollution than any other industry.[5] These animals produce 130 times the waste of the entire human population of the United States, eighty-seven thousand pounds of waste per second.[6] Much of the waste from factory farms—which contains high levels of toxic chemicals from pesticides, herbicides, antibiotics, hormones, and other pharmaceuticals—flows into and contaminates streams, rivers, and oceans.

3. Water use: More than half the water consumed in the United States is used to raise animals for food.[7] It takes eight thousand five hundred gallons of water to produce a pound of beef,[8] but only twenty-five gallons to produce a pound of wheat.[9] A vegan diet requires three hundred gallons of water per day; a meat eating diet requires more than four thousand gallons of water per day.[10]

4. Oceans: The world's oceans are being emptied of life. Most of the fish and other sea creatures caught annually are not eaten directly by humans but are fed to livestock. It may take twelve pounds of grain to make one pound of beef, but it also takes a hundred pounds of fish to make one pound of beef. It takes fifty pounds of wild fish to raise one farm-raised salmon.[11]

---

[5] Frances Moore Lappe, Diet for a Small Planet (New York: Ballantine Books, 1975) 22.
[6] Ed Ayres, "Will We Still Eat Meat?," Time Magazine 8 Nov. 1999.
    Also see the U.S. Senate Committee on Agriculture's 1997 report Animal Waste Pollution in America: An Emerging National Problem.
[7] Frances Moore Lappe, Diet for a Small Planet, 10th ed. (New York: Ballantine Books, 1982) 69.
[8] Matt Moore, "Institute Warns of Possible Water Shortage," Associated Press. 20 Apr. 2004.
[9] Robbins, The Food Revolution, 236.
[10] John Robbins, Diet for a New America (Tiburon, CA: HJ Kramer, 1998) 367.
[11] Paul Watson, "Consider the Fishes," VegNews March-April 2003: 27.

5. Land: Of all the agricultural land in the United States, eighty percent is used to raise animals for food and the crops to feed them.[12] That's forty-five percent of the total landmass in the United States.

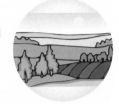

6. Deforestation: Our wild forests, which are habitats for wild animals, are disappearing. An acre of land disappears every eight seconds, cleared to grow crops to feed confined animals in factory farms.[13] These crops are heavily contaminated with herbicides and pesticides, and in many cases these plants have been genetically engineered and contain genetically modified organisms (GMOs) that infiltrate our ecosystem.

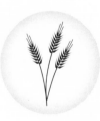

7. Crops: In the United States, eighty percent of the corn and more than ninety-five percent of the oats grown are fed to animals raised for food.[14] Most of the soybeans grown in the world are not used to make tofu or soymilk for people but are fed to livestock. Most of this feed has been genetically manipulated and is heavily laden with herbicides and pesticides.

8. Fossil fuel depletion: Over one-third of all fossil fuels used in the United States go to raise animals for food.[15] The war in the Middle East, the war for oil, is being fought to fuel the meat and dairy industries in the United States. Agriculture accounts for more than twice as much of the United States energy budget as the military.[16]

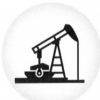

---

[12] Kenneth S. Krupa and Marlowe Vesterby, "Major Uses of Land in the United States," Statistical Bulletin No. 973 (United States Department of Agriculture, 1997).

[13] Will Tuttle, Ph.D, The World Peace Diet (New York: Lantern Books, 2005) 185.

[14] H. J. Maidenburg, "The Livestock Population Explosion," New York Times 1 Jul. 1973. Jane E. Brody, Give Us This Day (Arnold Press, 1975) 222.

[15] Jolinda Hackett, "What Does Eating Meat Have to do with Fossil Fuels?," About.com 19 Aug. 2008 <http://www.about.com/od/vegetarianvegan101/f/fossilfuels.htm?p=1> .

[16] Regional Farm and Food Project Oct. 2006 <http://www.farmandfood.org/newscommentary/articles_past/News_oct06.htm>.

We are depriving ourselves and future generations of fresh water, clean air, and a toxin-free world. Our human technology is an extension of our unenlightened minds, which do not grasp the interconnectedness of life. As a result, we are rapidly contaminating all living things, present and future, by raising animals for food.

When left alone, undomesticated animals may not possess the technological skills and tools that we have, but they may have something more vital that we do not: an innate intelligence and awareness of how to successfully coexist on Earth in the long term. Our environment is not becoming contaminated and barren because of wild animals. It is not because of them that we cannot drink from our rivers, lakes, and streams. Animals are naturally able to live with this planet and one another in ways that are sustainable and do not poison the air, soil, and water, or destroy the habitats of other beings. We, on the other hand, are destroying everyone else and ourselves with our destructive lack of awareness. Currently, the atrocities committed against animals in the name of human progress are the most important issues facing us all. With careful investigation, we will discover that most other issues plaguing us—from health crises to environmental woes to wars fought over land and oil—stem from it. Perhaps if we were to reverse our ways of relating to animals as mere things and instead began listening to them and observing how they live in harmony with the planet, we could learn some valuable lessons.

Yoga serves to awaken and remind us that we do know how to live in harmony with life. When we rediscover our own wildness, the shackles of our present culture will fall away, and we will find ourselves liberated from pretense and uncertainty. Yoga reveals to us the constraints and toxicity of our present culture. Yoga can show us the path to a renewed way of life and, ultimately, a way for us to stay alive.

In a larger context asana refers to our relationship to the Earth, which includes the environment as well as all beings. But as is true of all "life" philosophies, there are both esoteric and exoteric components that must be considered in order to develop deeper understanding of what it means to be alive. Yoga philosophy teaches that the reality we perceive as outside us is actually a reflection of what is inside us. This being so, the physical practice of asana allows us to deeply investigate, on a causal level, our relationship with the Earth and all other beings. It is through the investigation of our own body and mind that we discover within ourselves tendencies that we now see outside ourselves and want to change. Asana practice is indeed a very physical practice that respects the knowledge stored in the body and views the body not merely as something that carries the head around.

We cannot really "do" yoga, because Yoga is our natural state of being. Yoga refers to that enlightened state of living in harmony with all of existence. What we can do are certain practices that may reveal to us where we are resisting that natural state. Once these resistances are revealed or brought to the light of our conscious awareness, we have a better chance of letting them go. Asana practice, like meditation, is in essence a means of "letting go" of that which we are not, to reveal who we truly are. This is why you can't "do" it. You can only let go and allow it. When the resistances arise, we recognize and perceive them for what they truly are, or we might say, "where they are coming from."

Our bodies don't lie: they tell the story of our past. Our bodies are made up of the residue of all of our past unresolved karmas. For something to be a yoga practice, it must help us purify these karmas. The practice of asana is a yoga practice because it allows us to resolve past relationships with others and clarify our perception of ourselves.

Therapeutically, asana has the power to heal emotional traumas and put the personality back into order, so that we may function as happier, better-adjusted individuals. Essentially, however, the practice is designed to bring the individual beyond the healing of the body and mind and into a greater realization of the Self as whole, existing as a part of cosmic, eternal reality.

While we are engaged in certain asanas, particular physical and mental feelings arise. These feelings provide valuable insight into the nature of our personality—self. Ultimately, through the practice of asana, one can resolve the small self into the experience of the transcendent Self. This is possible because each time we engage in a particular asana, whether a standing pose like *trikonasana*, a forward bend like *paschimottanasana*, a twisting pose like *ardha matsyendrasana*, a backbend like *dhanurasana*, or an inversion like *sarvangasana*, we energetically relive past karmic experiences that have been stored in the cells and tissues of our physical body. (Refer to Appendix 3, *Yoga on the Mat*.)

Asana practice stimulates healing on many levels. Yes, it can help to heal injuries and bring strength and flexibility to muscles and joints, but, spiritually, the practice of asana can release us from *avidya*, which means ignorance of who we really are. The practice of asana releases *pranic* (life-giving) energy, allowing it to flow through heretofore-blocked subtle channels. When these channels flow with energy, we start to heal the disease of disconnection and begin to experience ourselves as much more than our physical body or personality self. We begin to experience ourselves as cosmic. What does that mean? It means we start to experience ourselves as part of a great whole, an interconnected eternal reality that transcends time and space. Wow! That's trippy!

Since yoga is a very practical science, before tripping out into the psychedelic mind-blowing reality of cosmic oneness, let us first look into the reality of relative experience: the day-to-day here and now. After all, there is truth to the ancient alchemical precept "as above so below." To be free and make it to heaven, we must make heaven here on Earth. There is actually no other place to go but here. Everything we need to expand our consciousness is all right here and now. Asana is the key that can open up the doorway to the adventure waiting for us inside our own bodies, where our past, present, and future reside. By freeing our bodies of negative karmas (negative thoughts, words, and deeds), we awaken to the body as a potential vehicle for the Divine.

The Divine refers to that which is whole—that which is holy. When we are whole, we are able to become an instrument for peace, not destruction, because our actions arise out of the personal experience of the interconnectedness of all beings and things. Through our practice of asana we build a holy (whole) body. As we free our bodies from fear, jealousy, and anger, we lift these negative emotions from the planetary atmosphere—which is, after all, only a reflection of what's going on inside us.

The actual physical substance of our bodies is derived from the food we eat. What or even whom we eat is decided by how we perceive and relate to others. When Patanjali tells us that if we want enlightenment we should relate to others in a mutually beneficial way, he implies that we should not view others as objects to be used by us—if, that is, we truly want enlightenment. When reflected upon in this way, the sutra *sthira-sukham asanam* (PYS II.46) provides valuable insight into how to improve our relationships with the other animals with whom we share this planet. The asana practice we do on and off the mat provides us with profound opportunities to heal the planet and evolve our human consciousness.

If we are to survive as a species, we must make the transition from a culture based on slavery, exploitation, violence, and death to a way of life based on kindness, peace, harmony, and wholeness. The practice of yoga holds within it the means to dismantle our present culture and give us the know-how to build a new way of life. What could be a better place to start than with the question "What shall we eat today?"

Eating is the most fundamental basis for our life as it creates and maintains our physical body, without which we would have no life. The choice to eat a vegetarian/vegan diet will do more to revolutionize our bodies, minds, and spirit and bring about world peace than any other single act, because it powerfully effects change in the outside world through enacting that change from deep within our own bodies. Such change will put into motion a profound planetary revolution, because it makes other-centeredness, not self-centeredness, the number-one priority. Up until this point in history, we have been members of a culture that gives priority to self-centeredness. For thousands of years, the enslaving and exploitation of animals has escalated and continued unquestioned, but now we are questioning. We are at the brink of a new level of consciousness that considers the well-being of the whole, not just a privileged few.

Asana refers to our connection to the Earth and other beings. When we allow ourselves to delve deeper into the meaning of asana, we realize the power this ancient practice has to heal the global crisis we are facing. Asana provides us a way to heal ourselves from the disease of disconnection, through healing our relationships with others. When we feel physically, emotionally, mentally, and spiritually connected to nature and all other beings, the greater global healing can begin.

The Hopi Elders tell us that we have passed the eleventh hour (a time of reckoning) and that *now* is the hour. Therefore, we should deeply consider all of our relationships, including what or whom we are eating, and where and with whom we are living. The Hopi wisely tell us, "At this time in history, we are to take nothing personally, least of all ourselves, for the moment we do, our spiritual growth and journey come to a halt."

What could it mean to take oneself personally in such a way that causes one's spiritual growth to stop? Our culture is essentially a domineering, herding culture. It is based on the enslavement of others, primarily other animal nations. It encourages us to seek self-gratification at the expense of others, even at the expense of the greater Earth community, mistakenly assuming that we can exist outside that community. The separation of spirit and body and of humanity and nature are results of the notion that the Earth belongs only to human beings. This ignorance (*avidya*) and egotism (*asmita*) lead to low self-esteem, and leave us feeling that what we do as individuals has little bearing on the whole. This feeling of insignificance represents the "personal" delusion that the Hopi Elders describe as the ultimate hindrance to our spiritual advancement.

Through communal yoga practice, as we experience the wonder of breathing together in a variety of ways, Self-confidence arises. Through chanting mantras and prayers, adding our voices to the choir, a greater sense of well-being develops. When we practice asana together, rhythmically moving in tune with breath and intention, we overcome debilitating estrangement, as we feel a part of a greater community. This unifying experience comes from a deep-rooted space of expansive yet inclusive consciousness, where all of existence is connected and pulsating with the joy of this wholeness, or holiness. The realization of unity is joyful and cannot be attained through hard struggle (working against something), but only through holy celebration.

Holy celebration is inclusive, as it embraces the whole community. Not one of us is an isolated case. Every action has tremendous impact upon all of creation. We must take responsibility for our behavior by looking into the possible outcome of our every exhaled breath, word spoken, and action taken, asking ourselves, "Is this contributing to the happiness and well-being of the greater community?" This, truly, is the key to unlocking our potential, making a boundless future on this Earth possible. If it is not, then have the courage to recognize that it is not a holy celebration, because it does not include the whole. Stop holding your breath and get yourself in tune. Breathe with one another, dismantling our present master/slave culture, and find a new way of living, based in the universal, unifying musical language of rhythm, harmony, and partnership.

The Hopi Elders inspire us to pulsate with the global community when they encourage: "The time of the lone wolf is over—gather yourselves! Banish the word *struggle* from your attitude and your vocabulary. All that you do now must be done in a sacred manner and in celebration. We are the ones we have been waiting for!"

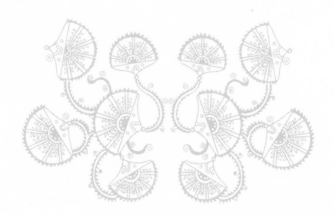

Chapter 2

AHIMSA

Nonharming

Who will be the happiest person?
The one who brings happiness to others.
—SWAMI SATCHIDANANDA

Three things in human life are important.
The first is to be kind, the second is to be kind, and
the third is to be kind.
—HENRY JAMES

Ahimsa means "nonharming." What happens when you practice ahimsa long enough to become established in it?

ahimsa-pratishthayam tat-sannidhau vaira-tyagah PYS II.35
When you stop harming others, others will cease to harm you.

ahimsa: nonharming, nonviolence
pratishthayam: being established or grounded in
tat: (in) that
sannidhau: presence
vaira: hostility
tyagah: give up, abandon

IN THE YOGA SUTRAS, PATANJALI GIVES US FIVE RECOMMENDATIONS, called *yamas*, for how we should treat others if we want to attain Yoga—the realization of the oneness of being. The first yama is *ahimsa*, which means "nonharming."

Patanjali says that if you are seeing a multitude of others and not One, then first and foremost, don't hurt them! The yamas are directives for how we should relate to others, not ourselves. Nonetheless, some contemporary yoga teachers interpret ahimsa as a directive not to harm yourself. "Don't be aggressive in your asana practice; be kind to your body," they say. Or else, "Don't restrict your diet with extremes like vegetarianism; it might harm you."

If Patanjali had been recommending ahimsa as a way of treating oneself, he would have included it in his list of *niyamas*, the observances one should maintain in regard to oneself. The five niyamas are: *saucha* (cleanliness), *santosha* (contentment), *tapas* (discipline), *svadhyaya* (study), *ishvara-pranidhana* (devotion). None of these niyamas conflicts with ethical vegetarianism, while the yamas all support it. Not harming yourself is a *result* of the practice of ahimsa, but if you limit your practice of ahimsa to being kind to yourself, you will deny yourself the ultimate benefit of yoga practice, which is enlightenment. The fact that Patanjali placed ahimsa as the first yama, and not among the personal observances, or niyamas, seems vitally significant. So much of the violence we see in the world today seems to be out of our control, but what we choose to eat is very much within our control.

We cannot change the suffering that has already happened in our lives, but future suffering can and should be avoided. A benefit of not causing others to suffer is that we will eventually, but inevitably, become free from suffering. We may mistakenly think that to refrain from harming another brings benefit only to that other, and not to ourselves. We often view extending kindness to animals as a form of charity. Many nonvegetarians may even look upon vegetarians as depriving themselves of enjoyment by refraining from eating meat. But when you understand how karma works and how yoga works, you begin to realize that how you treat others *now* determines how much suffering or joy you experience in your future.

In the case of eating meat, fish, and dairy products, the suffering may occur relatively quickly in the form of health problems like heart disease, stroke, or cancer. But most often the karmic seeds of violence, like all seeds, take time to gestate, sprout, and grow. One may not see the results of one's harmful actions right away. In fact, the negative seeds we plant now may not come to fruition until future lifetimes. There is no such thing as "instant karma." If there were, eating a hamburger would cause a person to drop dead.

Through the practice of yoga and ethical vegetarianism, we can realize that we were meant to live in harmony with all the other animals and all of life. We come to know that our physical bodies function better without having to instill fear into others and to kill them, and that there is no nutrient that we need that we can't get directly from plant sources or from sunlight. We will come to recognize that our old bodies can be transformed and become light and whole—holy bodies, used as vehicles to bring peace. We can truly become the peace we wish to see in the world, and all beings will rejoice in our presence and not fear and run away from us.

Nonharming is essential to the yogi, because it creates the kind of karma that leads to eternal joy and happiness. According to the universal law of karma, if you cause harm to others, you will suffer the painful consequences of your actions. The yogi, realizing this, tries to cause the least amount of harm and suffering to others possible.

Compassion is an essential ingredient of ahimsa. Through compassion, you begin to see yourself in other beings. This helps you refrain from causing harm to them. Developing compassion does something more that is of special interest to the yogi. It trains the mind to see beyond outer differences of form. You begin to catch glimpses of the inner essence of other beings, which is happiness. You begin to see that every single creature desires happiness.

To develop compassion, examine the motives behind your actions. Are they selfish or unselfish? Proclaiming that it is right to eat meat because it makes you healthier, for example, is *himsic*, or harmful, because it is an action stemming from a selfish motive. When you recognize that cows, pigs, and chickens, as well as all animals raised for food, want happiness just like you do, you recognize kindred souls. The distinction between you and other beings wears thin as awareness begins to dawn.

In truth, we all share consciousness, and harm inflicted on one being (be it animal or human) is felt by all, sooner or later. Some meat eaters like to advance the argument that vegetables have feelings, too, so what is the difference between eating chickens or carrots? The answer is simple: Patanjali gives ahimsa as a *practice*, meaning you do your best to cause the least amount of harm. The yogi strives to cause the least amount of harm possible, and it is clear that eating a vegetarian diet causes the least harm to the planet and all creatures.

Generally speaking, the "disease of disconnection" plagues the human condition. As a species, we are not at ease with ourselves—with our bodies, with our minds, or our feelings—nor are we at ease with others, whether human beings or other animals. We can be nervous, competitive, fearful, or worried. We crave respect and approval while simultaneously seeking dominance and power. We certainly aren't at ease with our environment and are constantly altering it to suit our needs or, more often, our desires, with little regard for how our actions impact others or the Earth. This "dis-ease" causes all sorts of problems. We are destroying ourselves, other animal species, and the planet in a misguided quest to find happiness or ease of being.

By enslaving other animals and abusing them through lifelong torture and degradation, we deprive them of freedom and happiness. How can we ourselves hope to be free or happy when our own lives are rooted in depriving others of the very thing we say we value most in life—the freedom to pursue happiness? If you want to bring more peace and happiness into your own life, the method is to stop causing violence and unhappiness in the lives of others.

We tell our children that "might is not right," yet we throw that idea out the window when it comes to the everyday reality of using might to torture, humiliate, and kill the enslaved and confined animals we raise for food.

maitryadishu balani PYS III.24
Through kindness, strength comes.

maitri: friendliness
adishu: et cetera (compassion, kindness)
balani: strength, power

This is a radical concept because it challenges our enculturation, which tells us that strength comes from weakening another. The fork can be a powerful weapon of mass-destruction or a tool to lead a movement of peaceful coexistence. Eating a compassionate vegetarian diet will stop war, create peace in one's body, peace with the animal nations, and peace on Earth.

Indeed, it is very radical to be a vegetarian during these times! As Ingrid Newkirk reminds us: "Never be afraid of seeming radical. All the best people in history have always been radical." The word *radical*, like the word *radish*, derives from the root word *rad*, meaning "root." A radical is someone who attempts to dig to the root of a situation. Yogis have always been radical and were even considered heretical because Yoga philosophy says a mediator or priest is not necessary—*you* are a direct line to God. Yogis search for the root causes because they understand that effective change can only occur if you change a course of action from the causal point. Failure to understand this is why so many "liberating" revolutions of the past never elicited long-lasting positive change; they only dealt with surface symptoms, not the root causes of social and cultural problems.

If we are to discover lasting solutions for our contemporary problems, we should look at the circumstances that might have led to those problems. History shows us that the enslavement of animals served as the model for human slavery. First animals were enslaved and exploited, and then it was not a far leap to begin treating humans "like animals" by enslaving and exploiting them as well.

In ancient India, the cow was economically essential. The word for cow became synonymous with many other terms used to describe the values of a culture founded upon the exploitation of animals, primarily cattle. The goddess of nature, for instance, was called "the perfect cow" because she provided abundance for her worshipers. So people came to look upon nature as existing to be used and exploited. Cow herders from ancient times to the present have viewed the cow's existence as a means to provide human beings the four M's: milk, meat, manure, and money.

In our quest for peace, it is valuable to recognize that the ancient wars in our culture's history were fought over disputes about animal ownership and the land needed to confine, graze, and grow crops to feed those animals. Interestingly, the Sanskrit word for war is *gavya*, literally meaning "the desire to fight for more cattle," and *gavishti* means "to be desirous of a fight." Both words come from the root *gav* or *go*, which means "cow." The domestication (enslaving) of cows led to war.

Yogis seek real and lasting liberation from suffering. The Sanskrit term *jivanmukti* reveals the philosophical idea that such liberation is possible even for a person who still has a physical body, rather than only after the body is shed. *Jiva* means "individual soul," and *mukti* means "liberation." Together, the words describe a liberated soul, a person who perceives him- or herself not as a separate individual, but as holy: one who is part of the whole of creation.

The *jivanmukta* experiences liberation—absolute freedom from all states of confinement and suffering—and wishes this for all beings. In Tibetan Buddhism, we find a similar idea in the concept of the *bodhisattva*: one who lives for the benefit of others and finds the highest joy in the happiness and liberation of others. Yoga means liberation. Slavery is contrary to liberation. We ourselves can never be free while taking away freedom from others. Through the practice of yoga, we begin to recognize ourselves as inseparable from the whole and realize that whatever we do to others we ultimately do to ourselves.

Pratishthayam means "to become well established or grounded in a certain practice." If we want to live in a less violent world, then we will have to give up violence ourselves. As we become less violent, the world around us becomes less violent. We cannot demand something that we ourselves are not willing to embody.

I once spoke to a well-known yoga teacher, who is not a vegetarian and who had told his students that vegetarianism isn't an important aspect of the practice of yoga, about the subject of *ahimsa-pratishthayam* (being established in ahimsa). In a public statement at a yoga conference, he had said that it was not necessary to be a vegetarian in order to be established in ahimsa. I asked him if he felt that a person could kill and eat an animal without causing the animal harm, which would be the only logical support for his statement. Instead of answering my question directly, he asked me if I thought that Jesus and the Buddha were enlightened beings, and went on to tell me that neither of them were vegetarians. "How do you know that they were not vegetarians?" I asked. The reality is that no one knows for sure what they ate or didn't eat, but we certainly do know what *we* have been eating. We also know for sure whether we are living a peaceful, easeful life or one filled with violence and hostility.

Yoga is said to be the perfection of action by the removal of selfish motivation. Yogis use the world they live in and the way in which they interact with the world as a vehicle for transformation. A vegan diet is an informed, intelligent, and conscious way to act peacefully and selflessly each time we make a choice, because it takes into consideration the well-being of others as well as of ourselves.

The practice of yoga builds inner confidence. As we become more Self-confident, we become less fearful. We become less self-absorbed, and our ability to feel life all around allows us to hear what life is trying to communicate to us through nature. Speaking to us through the animals, trees, water, and air, the message is simple yet profound: All of life is interconnected. What we do to others affects us all. When we begin to feel this, we can free ourselves from the false idea that the Earth belongs to us and instead use our lives to benefit others. In turn, we will become happy as we discover that the best way to uplift our own lives is to do all we can to uplift the lives of others. When we become well established in ahimsa, we live in such a way that all hostility ceases in our presence. Others will not harm us. They won't feel any animosity toward us or even think harmful thoughts about us. They will have no need to fear us. Animals will not cower or shake in our presence or fearfully run away from us. As we rid ourselves of violent tendencies, we purify the atmosphere surrounding us, which is but a projection of our inner ground of being.

Chapter 3

SATYA

Telling the Truth

---

*If people knew the truth about how badly animals are
treated in today's factory farms, if people knew how
completely confined and immobilized these creatures are
for their entire lives, if people knew how severe and
unrelenting is the cruelty these animals are forced to
endure, there would be change. If people knew, but too
many of us choose to look the other way, to keep the veil
in place, to remain unconscious and caught in the cultural
trance. That way we are more comfortable. That way is
convenient. That way, we don't have to risk too much. This
is how we keep ourselves asleep.*
—John Robbins

Satya means "truthfulness." What happens when one becomes
established in truth?

satya-pratishthayam kriya-phalashrayatvam PYS II.36
*When one does not defile one's speech with lies, the words one
says are listened to and acted upon in a positive and immediate
manner. The speaker will be able to say what they mean. What
one says comes true.*

satya: truth
pratishthayam: being established or grounded in
kriya: purifying action
phala: fruit, fruition, to come to pass
ashrayatvam: dependency

TREACHERY AND DECEIT WERE THE METHODS USED INITIALLY, thousands of years ago, to "domesticate" animals: kill the parents, steal the baby, raise the orphan as if it were your own child. Thus, the baby bonds to you and grows up thinking it is part of your family. In this way, animals become dependent upon you and trust you. You can easily exploit them—shear them, milk them, use them to make more babies. Then, when you have exhausted their usefulness to you, you kill them and—the final humiliation—eat them. This master/slave relationship began by deceiving baby animals and continues to this day.

When the natural bond that occurs between child and parent is dissolved, the child is not able to develop in a healthy way, and physical and psychological breakdowns are inevitable. The child remains dysfunctional, with a distorted perception of itself and others. This vulnerability makes it more easily manipulated by its oppressors. It is easier to manipulate others when you take away their personhood and see them as objects.

Life on a farm has never been a happy, healthy family experience for the animals. Even before the onset of factory farms, a farm was a place to raise and harvest animals. In agriculture, seeds are planted with the intention of reaping crops. Farm animals are treated like vegetables—as if they had the feelings of vegetables. Farms are breeding facilities, where rape and manipulation are common daily procedures. Farm animals are not allowed to develop normal relationships with others of their kind. The cow, pig, or ewe for instance will never actually have the chance to have a relationship with the male whose seed will father her children. She never even gets to have a relationship with the children she will give birth to. In most cases, she isn't even allowed to see or to touch her babies. She is kept chained to a stall looking straight ahead or, in the case of pigs, strapped down on her side on a concrete floor, immobilized as she gives birth and for the short time that she nurses her piglets.

The consumer is not told the truth about where food comes from. Instead, we are told lies. The meat and dairy industry spends millions of dollars on advertising to deceive us. Because the meat and dairy industries form the foundation of our economic system, government agencies also don't want the public to know. There are laws now protecting the animal user industries from citizen scrutiny. It is becoming harder and harder for animal rights groups to gain access into factory farms or slaughterhouses to film or take photographs. The few pictures and pieces of film footage that do exist and are available for public view are very threatening to the animal user industries. Why? Because in our culture "seeing is believing," and these films and pictures show the truth, a truth that once seen is impossible to deny. We have a worldwide culture of denial when it comes to our treatment of animals. No one wants to talk about it. In fact it is considered taboo to speak of it, as it may spoil one's appetite.

When advertising is employed to sell meat, milk, and eggs, pictures of happy animals enjoying family life on the farm are used: calves grazing beside their mothers in lush green fields or cute fluffy baby chicks surrounding a doting mother hen in a country barnyard. The truth is that in factory farms, and in farms in general, mothers are never allowed to be with their babies. Images like this are false advertising. Although in our hearts we know the truth about how food animals are being used, we lie to ourselves. We perpetuate this untruth when we lie to our children and fail to encourage them to investigate the truth.

The more we lie to others, the more others will lie to us. Eventually, it becomes quite normal to communicate through lying, never really saying what we mean or doing what we say.

Advertising and various media use lies to keep us convinced that we must continue to enslave animals, to use and exploit them, and to eat their meat. This is a form of lying, a violation of the power of speech that destroys any chance of creating an atmosphere of truthfulness, or satya. This fragmentation of body, mind, and speech prevents the development of *dharana*, the ability of the mind to concentrate, and ultimately blocks the ability to meditate and merge with blissful transcendental reality. The ability to concentrate is a difficult enough practice for most people, regardless of whether or not they are vegetarians. Meat eaters who try to meditate have to deal with that obstacle, not to mention the paranoia and fear they experience as a result of terrorizing others.

Some meat eaters say they are peaceful people and would never hurt anyone—they didn't kill the animal; they're just eating what is convenient. This type of thinking is an example of how disempowered and disconnected most of the carnivorous members of our culture feel. They have been convinced that what they do doesn't really matter in the larger scheme of things. After all, it is only my lunch—just a piece of ham between two slices of bread; what harm could that do? The fact is that when we buy the meat of an animal, we are the ones who have signed his or her death sentence. When a hit man is paid to murder someone, should we view the person who hired him as innocent and put the blame solely on the hired gun? If we are buying and eating meat and dairy products, then the slaughterhouse workers, meat packers, and factory farm workers are all working for us. If everyone in the world woke up tomorrow and refused to buy meat and dairy products they would no longer be lucrative industries, which is the only reason that they exist.

Part of the process of transitioning into living more honestly is to hold yourself accountable for the things you do. When we stop blaming others for our actions, we take a giant step toward freeing ourselves from low self-esteem, which arises through continuously relinquishing our decision-making power to others.

I am very close with a family whom I have known for years. I have seen the children grow up. The parents have always respected my veganism, and when I arrive for a visit, the whole family adopts a vegan diet for at least the time I am with them. Normally they aren't vegans and eat meat. One summer when I was visiting, one of the children, who was then a teenager, asked me why I was a vegan. I replied that I wanted to contribute to peace on this planet and not more violence. "So do I," he exclaimed. "You know me; I'm a very peaceful person, but I do eat meat. What does eating meat have to do with peace?"

"Eating animals is a violent act," I replied.

"Only if you kill the animal," he argued, "and I don't kill animals. I would never kill an animal or go hunting or hurt anyone. I just eat them, and someone else kills them."

"But you are the one paying for someone else to kill them. Doesn't that make you responsible?" I asked him.

"No," he replied, "because I don't buy the groceries. My parents do, not me."

This is not an isolated incident. Such feelings are commonplace in our hierarchical, structured societies. Accountability for one's actions is less important than doing what we are told or obediently going along with the crowd and never questioning. We are told over and over again that the actions of individuals are not important to the whole scheme.

The Perils of Obedience

PSYCHOLOGIST STANLEY MILGRAM CONDUCTED A FAMOUS EXPERIMENT in obedience at Yale University in the 1960s. It was a study of how obedience, as a deeply ingrained behavior in our culture, can override ethics. The experiment measured the willingness of study participants to obey an authority figure, who instructed them to perform acts that conflicted with their personal conscience.

In his experiment, two people come to a psychology laboratory to take part in a study. One of them is designated a "teacher," the other a "learner." The experimenter explains that the study is concerned with the effects of punishment on learning. The learner is conducted into a room and strapped into a chair with what appears to be an electrode attached to his wrist. He is told that he will be read lists of simple word pairs by the teacher and that he will then be tested on his ability to remember the second word of a pair when he hears the first one again. Whenever he makes an error, the teacher will administer electric shocks of increasing intensity by pulling on a lever.

The teacher is a genuinely naïve subject. The learner is actually an actor who receives no shock at all but pretends to. The learner sitting in the chair is in full view of the teacher. When the learner begins to miss words, the teacher pulls the lever to administer a shock. When the actor/learner would convulse and appear to be really suffering, and even screaming, the teacher would inevitably turn to the experimenter and ask to stop the experiment. The experimenter would always respond by insisting that the teacher continue with the experiment. The actor/learner would express pain more dramatically, and the teacher would again turn to the experimenter to ask if the experiment should be halted. The experimenter would insist firmly that the teacher must complete the experiment.

Most of the subjects who participated in the experiment continued to shock the learner even while protesting to the experimenter that they felt what they were doing was unethical. They obeyed the experimenter in spite of their own feelings.

The experiments began in July 1961, three months after the start of the trial of Nazi war criminal Adolf Eichmann. Milgram said that he devised his experiment to question whether it was possible that Eichmann and his accomplices were just following orders.

"The question arises," he wrote in the preface to his book, *Obedience to Authority*, "as to whether there is any connection between what we have studied in the laboratory and the forms of obedience we so deplored in the Nazi epoch. The essence of obedience consists in the fact that a person comes to view himself as the instrument for carrying out another person's wishes, and he therefore no longer regards himself as responsible for his actions."[17]

"Ordinary people, simply doing their jobs, and without any particular hostility on their part, can become agents in a terrible destructive process. Moreover, even when the destructive effects of their work become patently clear, and they are asked to carry out actions incompatible with fundamental standards of morality, relatively few people have the resources needed to resist authority."[18]

"Even Eichmann was sickened when he toured the concentration camps, but he had only to sit at a desk and shuffle papers. At the same time, the man in the camp who actually dropped the Zyklon B into the gas chambers was able to justify his behavior on the ground that he was only following orders from above. Thus there is a fragmentation of the total human act. No one man decides to carry out the evil act and

---

[17] Stanley Milgram, <u>Obedience to Authority</u> (New York: Harper Collins, 1974) xviii.
[18] Stanley Milgram, "The Perils of Obedience," <u>Harper's Magazine</u> 1974.

is confronted with its consequences. The person who assumes full responsibility for the act has evaporated. Perhaps this is the most common characteristic of socially organized evil in modern society."[19] In Milgram's experiment, sixty-five percent of the people tested did administer the highest voltage of electric shocks.

Interestingly, there was another experiment conducted during the early sixties, with rhesus monkeys (also known as macaques) instead of human subjects. The majority of the monkeys refrained from operating a device for securing food if it caused another monkey to suffer an electric shock.[20] One description of the experiment reads: "In a laboratory setting, macaques were fed if they were willing to pull a chain and electrically shock an unrelated macaque whose agony was in plain view through a one-way mirror. Otherwise, they starved. After learning the ropes the monkeys frequently refused to pull the chain; in one experiment only thirteen percent would do so—eighty-seven percent preferred to go hungry. One macaque went without food for nearly two weeks rather than hurt its fellow. Macaques who had themselves been shocked in previous experiments were even less willing to pull the chain. The relative social status or gender of the macaques had little bearing on their reluctance to hurt others.... By conventional human standards, these macaques—who have never gone to Sunday school, never heard of the Ten Commandments, never squirmed through a single junior high school civics lesson—seem exemplary in their moral grounding and their courageous resistance to evil."[21]

In their behavior toward animals, all men are Nazis; for the animals it is an eternal Treblinka.

—Isaac Bashevis Singer

---

[19] Milgram, Obedience to Authority, ii.
[20] Jules Masserman, M.D., William Terris, M.S., and Stanley Wechkin, Ph.D., "Altruistic Behavior in Rhesus Monkeys," American Journal of Psychiatry 121 (1964): 584-585.
[21] Carl Sagan and Ann Druyan, Shadows of Forgotten Ancestors (New York: Ballantine Books, 1992) 117.

Through the practices of yoga, we begin to connect to a place of conscience, which provides us with information about the possible outcome of our actions. To act from conscience is to act from independence—from being dependent inward. That place, which some call the heart, is our connection to the greater world or the greater heart. When we act out of conscience, our actions are never merely self-serving; they serve the whole. As the Milgram experiment shows, our cultural conditioning can be so strong that it disconnects us from our heart, leading to a feeling of disempowerment. We can become programmed to act in a way that is fragmented and not true to ourselves. To do something because everybody else does it is not a good enough reason. To do it because we believe God told us to do it is not a good enough reason either. To live by violence and then to deny that you do is to live a lie. Living a lie causes a deep fissure in the human psyche. Yoga seeks to heal that fissure.

One of the ways that you can tell if you are making progress in yoga, especially hatha yoga, is by observing your own voice. Through regular practice, you will find that you are able to adjust the volume and pitch of your voice so that you can be heard and understood, but most importantly, you will be able to say what you mean and mean what you say. When this happens, it is an indication that the disease of disconnection is beginning to be healed. You will be increasingly able to articulate with integrity from a place of deep universal connectedness rather than isolation.

It is thought of as quite normal these days for people to say one thing while thinking something else, and then do a contradictory third thing. One underlying cause of this symptom is that we have conditioned ourselves to disconnect from the reality of how we view and treat animals.

Most of us say we want peace, equality, and freedom for all, but our actions say something entirely different as we bite into a hamburger or order an ice-cream cone, wear a fur coat to an anti-war demonstration or serve hot dogs to our children. Once you become more aware, there's simply no way to not notice these everyday hypocrisies, these gaps in awareness justified by group behavior and the culture of dis-ease.

By contemplating these issues with sincerity, you will realize that they are just an outgrowth of our ancient animal slave-based culture, which surrounds all of us at every turn. This disconnection between one's feelings or heartfelt beliefs and what one says and does stems from a patriarchal herding culture as old as Babylon. It may be interesting to note that Sumer, considered the cradle of Western civilization, is where both the herding of animals and the development of written language originated. The Sumerian cuneiform tablets are among the oldest written literature existing. This vast litera-ture, mostly in poetic form, tells of man's conquest of animals and of nature and his move toward urban societies built upon a hierarchical system of government, religion, and economics based upon animal slavery.

For thousands of years, we have conditioned ourselves to do things that we know in our hearts are morally wrong; yet, we do them, because we have been told to do so by the authority figures in our lives. We have been told that life is hard, and that in some situations we simply must "buck up" and do them anyway, even though they are unpleasant—like killing animals. We live a double standard: We don't want to tell our children where their food is coming from and don't want to do the killing, but we don't question the lie at the core of our abusive treatment of animals. The truth is that we don't have to hurt them, kill them, or eat them to be happy, healthy, and wise, but in order to become aware of that we must de-condition ourselves and explore ways to live and act from a place of the heart. As Stanley Milgram suggests, "It may be that we are puppets—controlled by the strings of society. But at least we are puppets with perception, with awareness. And perhaps our awareness is the first step to our liberation."

In *The Animals Film*, the filmmaker asked random people on the street the question "Do you like animals?" One woman gave the very revealing answer: "Animals? I *love* animals!" Then he asked, "Do you eat animals?" The woman responded incredulously: "Eat animals? Yes. Doesn't everybody?" The filmmaker then asked: "But you said you loved animals. Is there a contradiction there?" To which the woman replied, "Well, I'd like to live by my principles, but I don't, 'cause we gotta eat, don't we?"

The industries that exploit animals create self-serving euphemisms to conceal the truth of their actions. A survey of your local supermarket will turn up such terms as "humanely slaughtered" and "raised according to animal welfare standards" on packages of meat and cartons of eggs. If you look up *humane* in a dictionary, you will find: characterized by compassion, sympathy, kindness, mercy, or consideration for other human beings or animals. If you look up *welfare*, you might find: concerned for another's health, happiness, and well-being.

These industries have become experts at what Tom Reagan refers to as "Humpty-Dumpty talk" in his book *Empty Cages*.[22] In Lewis Carroll's classic, *Through the Looking Glass*, when Alice comes across the egg, Humpty-Dumpty, they have a conversation in which Alice becomes frustrated with Humpty's way of defining things. He uses words to mean something totally different from what they actually mean. When Alice confronts him with this, he says, "When I use a word, it means just what I choose it to mean—neither more nor less."

We, in turn, use Humpty-Dumpty talk to lie to our children about what we are really feeding them, and they grow up learning that no one has to be honest about anything. They are given the message that denial, not honesty, is valued

---

[22] Tom Reagan, Empty Cages (Oxford: Rowman & Littlefield, 2004) 78.

and should be cultivated. We override our children's natural sense of compassion by showing them pictures on packages of meat of cute animals dressed up and happy, or cartoons of pigs eating ribs, cows offering ice-cream sundaes, or smiling burgers bouncing up and down in a burger-garden saying, "Eat me please!"

If we don't want to be taken in by the lies people tell us, we can begin to examine our own speech and ask ourselves if we are really saying what we mean. If we say we want peace on Earth, are we willing to do what is necessary to create it? Are we willing to speak truthfully at every turn and be honest with others and ourselves? This is difficult work, but once begun, it becomes easier with practice. It is, like yoga itself, a lifelong effort.

If we want others to speak well of us, are we willing to stop gossiping, judging, and blaming others? True or not, we humans tend to assume that we are superior to other animals because we have the ability to speak. Yet it has been observed by scientists that other animals can and do speak, but in languages that we cannot understand. All of nature communicates. Why is it that we cannot hear what she is saying? We want so much for others to hear us. Half the effort in speaking truthfully lies in listening well. Are we listening to the anguished cries of the animals in factory farms or the shrieks of the slaughtered?

If we grew up eating meat and dairy products, then our own bodies have been formed from animals whose voices we had a hand in silencing when they were locked away to cry on their own in lonely warehouses and had their throats cut at the time of slaughter. How might this have an impact upon our own ability to speak truthfully...and to be heard?

I have observed in my years of teaching yoga that many students are quite shy when it comes to speaking in public, let alone singing or chanting mantras. Shyness could be seen as a form of vanity because it exists when we are thinking of ourselves and our feelings and not the feelings of the people in front of us. It lacks empathy and comes from a deep self-consciousness and self-absorption, which stems from feeling separate.

Why do so many of us feel so shy? Musician and activist Michael Franti says that the biggest fear people have is the fear of having to speak in public and that fear is only second to the fear of having to sing in public. But why? Some people blame early childhood experiences; perhaps teachers, parents or siblings silenced them with harsh judgmental words like, "Shut up! You can't carry a tune," or "You're no Pavarotti or Elvis Presley!" These types of experiences are by no means rare in our culture but might be viewed as symptoms rather than causes.

If we look more deeply at some of our more indigenous human relatives who have not distanced themselves so far from nature and live more closely with wild animals, we find societies in which singing and dancing are considered normal everyday activities for every member of the tribe. Within so-called uncivilized tribal societies, singing and dancing is not a performance art or "dis-play" but is engaged in as actual play—a form of communication with life, rather than as a commodity to be taken to the market place. Have we traded our natural musical abilities, which would allow us to express ourselves freely or even wildly in song and dance, for a more domesticated version of ourselves?

Most of us unconsciously accept that our "civilized way" of life is better than the wild savage version. After all, we have been told this over and over again over countless lifetimes. We, in turn, pass on these unexamined assumptions to our children, unaware that we may be lying to them and to ourselves. We don't question the results of a ten-thousand-year-old war on animals, nature, and all that is wild. Yet our domesticated civilized life has been bought at great cost, not only to nature and the animals, but to us. As we have domesticated animals and robbed them of their wildness, we have become domesticated ourselves and lost our natural ability to be expressive and spontaneous. We have become nervous, neurotic, self-conscious, and—at the same time—vain and arrogant.

I once visited an animal sanctuary in South Carolina which rescues exotic animals from abusive situations in circuses, sideshows, theme parks, and the like, and provides them with a fairly safe haven. I say "fairly" because they are still captive, but at least they are spared the degradation of travel and performance. When I first arrived, the owner was very excited to give me a tour and introduce me to some of the lions, tigers, elephants, baboons, chimpanzees, zebras, bears, wolves, and mountain lions (to name but a few). He took me to the "nursery" to show me the babies and said, "My commitment is to, number one, help these animals get over their fear of humans and, number two, help them get over their fear of each other." The nursery was a fenced-in yard with a large barn attached. Every morning he brings all the babies together to play and returns them to their parents in the afternoon. I was immediately greeted by two five-month-old tigers, who ran to me, tumbling over themselves in the process. The tigers shared their play space with a baby mountain lion, a baby bear named Ursula, and Bambina, a gentle, big-eyed, two-month-old fawn. They all seemed to be quite chummy with one another, but that wasn't the most extraordinary thing that struck me as I sat on the ground surrounded by these furry children. It was the cacophony of voices: they all seemed to be speaking at once. From my perspective, it appeared that they were either in a continuous dialogue with one another, mumbling to themselves, or just talking and singing for the sake of it.

I was literally dumbstruck, as I had ignorantly assumed that all animals were basically mute and only let out a howl, bark, or meow on occasion, like the pet dogs and cats I had known (except for the Siamese cats I have had the privilege of living with, who normally do engage in lengthy conversation and commentary on life).

From this experience, I gained an insight about how our domestication of animals and its repression of all their natural tendencies might have led to a repression of their voices, causing them to become mute. The common practice used in all situations where there is slavery is to separate the babies from their parents while they are very young. The babies are not allowed to develop communication and speaking skills, as they would have if they had been allowed to be tutored by their parents. Wild animals, in contrast, talk a lot and without inhibition. Could there be a connection between how we have treated animals and our own inability to speak or sing freely?

In his book *Dominion*, Matthew Scully recounts, "I think of a fellow I know, in many respects devout and conscientious, who recently tried to shock me with a story about a laboratory (in Indiana, as I recall) where, to silence the yapping of some sixty dogs, the researchers cut out the vocal cords of each one. The dogs still try to bark, my colleague told me, as if relating some hilarious punchline, only it looks like someone has pressed the mute button, and now the scientists can go about their work in peace and quiet. Where does this spirit come from, that can laugh at such a thing?"[23]

As yoga practitioners, we come to a time in our lives when we begin to question whether what we have been told is true, including the assumptions we hold about ourselves and the world around us. The fact that you have begun a yoga practice is evidence that you have the courage to embark on a deep self-reflective quest. Through such self-reflection you will encounter blockages to your creativity and self-expression. It is during those crucial moments, while engaged in asana or meditation practice, that it is important not to harbor negative thoughts. Do not blame others or feel guilty, inadequate, or overwhelmed. Instead, allow the past karmic residue to arise, and let it go with each passing breath. Through steady practice

---

[23] Matthew Scully, Dominion: The Power of Man, the Suffering of Animals, and the Call to Mercy (New York: St. Martin's Press, 2002) 18.

(*abhyasa*), you will experience for yourself what is true, and all the lies you have been told, even those that you have told, will fade away in the light of the greater truth of your true potential.

As we embrace the practice of satya, our speech becomes purified, and we are able to fearlessly say what we mean and mean what we say. Others cease lying to us and begin to perceive us as people with integrity; they listen to us and take our words seriously. What we say comes true. As Mahatma Gandhi suggested, we "become the change we wish to see in the world."

Chapter 4

ASTEYA

Nonstealing

Yoga is that state where you are missing nothing.
—SHRI BRAHMANANDA SARASVATI

Asteya means "not to steal." What happens when one becomes established in asteya?

asteya-pratishthayam sarva-ratnopasthanam PYS II.37
When one stops stealing from others, prosperity
(material, mental, and spiritual) appears.

asteya: nonstealing
pratishthayam: being established or grounded in
sarva: all
ratna: jewels, money, wealth, prosperity
upasthanam: appear or approach

THE MEAT, DAIRY, AND FASHION INDUSTRIES ARE FOUNDED UPON stealing—stealing milk intended for a mother's new baby, stealing wool intended to keep someone warm, stealing skin and fur intended to be worn by the being who was born into that skin. To confine an animal for its entire life is to steal its life. To kill and eat animals is to steal their lives from them. The meat and dairy industries have successfully convinced us not to stop to think that animals may have their own purpose for living, which doesn't include being exploited and used up by us, their human enslavers.

Through the practice of yoga, you come to feel confident and develop a feeling of wholeness and completeness; you are not likely to feel deprived or "less than." People steal because they feel deprived. They try to make up for their deficits by depriving others. Our culture teaches us that if we have the money to pay for it, we can have it. We can own land or animals if we pay for them. We used to be able to own humans, if we paid for them, until we came to understand that human slavery is wrong. Now we are on the brink of realizing that enslaving animals is wrong.

Our present culture began roughly ten thousand years ago in Sumer, in the area currently known as Iraq. At that time, people began to domesticate animals. Dogs were the first, enslaved to help with hunting. Domestication is a polite way of describing enslavement. The first animals to be enslaved and exploited for food were sheep and goats. Before domestication, these animals were wild, living harmoniously with the rest of the natural world, as all wild animals know how to do. Once enslaved, the only purpose accorded to them by their captors was to be exploited by human beings, who controlled every aspect of their lives—deciding where they lived, whom they lived with, what they ate, and when they would die. These humans milked, sheared, bred, and ate the animals, considering them property. A person's wealth, power, and status came to be equated with the number of animals he owned and dominated.

After goats and sheep, cows were the next wild animals to be enslaved. It's funny, but most of us don't think of cows as once being wild animals. This shows something about how ingrained the notion of owning and eating animals has become. It seems normal to confine "barnyard animals," as if it has always been that way—as if they were born to live on farms as slaves. There is a growing movement of people today who feel that factory farms are wrong, but these people do not feel the same way about eating, milking, and exploiting animals in general. They would like to revert to the ideal of the small family-owned farm, not realizing that the small farm is, in essence, the factory farm on a smaller scale: a place where animals are fattened for slaughter. I feel that it is time for us to question the basic cultural assumption that animals exist as slaves to be exploited by us. If we ourselves want to get to the root cause of many of our problems today, we might start by critically examining the concept of the "farm."

Our English word *capital* comes from the Latin word *capita*, which means "head," referring to heads of cattle, sheep, or goats. The first capitalists fought wars over land and livestock, and we are still fighting.

According to Will Tuttle's book *The World Peace Diet*: "Livestock in the ancient herding cultures thus defined the value of gold and silver—food animals were the fundamental standard of wealth and power. This fact gives us insight into the political might of the ranching and dairy industries that continues to this day."[24] In fact, our modern-day term *stock market* is derived from the ancient practice of trading livestock as commodities.

In the way that organisms depend upon genes to keep their traits alive and embodied, a culture relies upon memes. A meme is an idea, behavior, style, or trend that spreads from person to person within a culture. When an idea or behavior becomes integrated into the minds and habits of a people, it becomes perceived unquestionably as "normal" and as "always having been this way—everybody does it." The exploitation of animals has become a meme. When you understand this, then you can take the first step in freeing yourself from the

---

[24] Tuttle, The World Peace Diet, 19.

propaganda of your culture. The practices of yoga help us to question these long-standing habits.

An important meme for our present culture is "the Earth belongs to us," implying that it is the right of human beings to exploit the Earth and all other beings. Yoga holds the power to dismantle our present culture and gives us the means to learn how to live harmoniously with nature. The word *exploitation* means "to treat with little regard for the welfare, benefit, or happiness of the other." We live in a culture in which most everyone agrees that it is okay to enslave animals and that it is okay to eat them. In fact, it is expected of us that we eat them, and it is considered strange to question this expectation.

The first mention of memes is found in ancient Sumerian texts, which are some of the oldest surviving texts of our present culture. In Sumerian mythology, the moon goddess, Inanna, daughter of the sun, was said to have stolen the memes from her father and used them to build a civilization. The first city she built was called Uruk, and it existed about 150 miles from present-day Baghdad. Archaeologists have discovered cuneiform tablets and cylindrical stone seals in this area. These seals are carved with pictures, some of which depict warriors in battle, shepherds, and cattle. Sumeria was a "land of milk and honey," an ancient meat-eating and milk-drinking civilization founded upon the enslavement of animals.

Our modern cities are based on the Sumerian meme, a way of life in which human beings' desires are given paramount importance and all other forms of life are perceived to exist primarily to be exploited by humans. Yoga has always existed in opposition to the rules, regulations, and cultural norms of the times in which it is practiced. The natural laws of beauty and harmony are the laws of the yogi. Yogis have always rejected the ways of civilization, with its degrading, imposing moral codes that, rather than respecting nature, are founded upon taming and manipulating her. Yoga is founded upon the love of nature and the pursuit of ecstasy. The yogi understands that there is an innate order to wildness and that liberation comes through the blessings of the Divine Goddess, who is Mother Nature. Shiva, who is said to have been the first teacher of yoga, is a wild man who lives in the forest with the animals. He is called *Pashupati*, which means "protector of the animals." You could say that Shiva was the first environmental/animal rights activist.

The moral codes of urban society would have us fear wildness, telling us it is chaotic. In truth, nature is anything but chaotic—she operates in a very organized fashion.

Ritual animal sacrifice was a product of a culture that kept domesticated animals as slaves to be used for exploitation. In India, yogis sought refuge in the forest, where they could live close to nature and keep their distance from such barbaric rites, preferring to seek communion with the Divine through direct means. Yogis were considered heretics for rejecting the idea that it was necessary to pay an intermediary to recite spells over the burning bodies of slain animal victims in order to connect with divinity. In *Gods of Love and Ecstasy: The Traditions of Shiva and Dionysus*, author Alain Danielou notes, "Throughout the course of history, urban and industrial societies—those exploiters and destroyers of the natural world—have been opposed to any ecological or mystical approach to the liberation of man and his happiness."[25]

Yoga is a tantric practice—worshiping the Goddess in the form of nature. Its methods align us with rather than oppose the forces of nature. Rejecting cultural pressure to despise the body and look upon it as animalistic, needing to be clothed and tamed, yogis value the physical body as a potential vehicle for direct ecstatic transcendental communion with the Divine.

In our present time, we may not think we are stealing from others when we eat meat and dairy products because we have been deluded into thinking that those others, the animal

---

[25] Alain Danielou, <u>Gods of Love and Ecstasy: The Traditions of Shiva and Dionysus</u> (Rochester: Inner Traditions, 1992) 16.

slaves, exist for our benefit and that if we pay at the super-market or the restaurant, then we are entitled to them. But the ultimate truth is that the animals never entered into any agreement to be bought and sold. We have been stealing their lives for our own selfish reasons. According to Patanjali, this is not conducive to our material, mental, and spiritual prosperity. This is how karma works. When we steal, we set into motion dire karmic consequences that affect our future well-being.

When someone says to me: "If people choose to eat meat, it is their business. We should not interfere, and we should be tolerant and accommodating of their dietary preferences," I have to say that whatever any of us does affects us all. When someone eats meat, it affects all of us because of the terrible environmental impact of the meat and dairy industries on the planet. By eating meat, we are not only stealing the lives and happiness of billions of animals, we are also stealing fresh water and clean air from future generations who will be born into this world.

At a yoga conference, I was having dinner with some colleagues when a certain dish was passed to me. Just before I was about to spoon out a portion onto my plate, someone remarked: "Oh, you probably won't want to eat that. It has butter and cheese in it." A yoga teacher sitting next to me asked: "What? You don't eat milk products? That's not very yogic, is it? What's wrong with milk? You can still be a vegetar-ian and drink milk, can't you? Isn't it more cruel to the cows not to milk them?"

I responded: "Milk is the fluid that comes from the breasts of a female cow when she is pregnant or has just given birth to a baby. The milk her body is producing is intended for her baby. I think it is in keeping with the principles of yoga to be kind (*ahimsa*) and not to steal from another (*asteya*) what is not intended for you."

"But," my friend continued, "drinking milk is better than eating flesh. At least no animal is being killed for you to drink milk."

"When her milk production drops," I replied, "every dairy cow ends up at the slaughterhouse."

"No, that's not true!" my friend emphatically stated.

"What do you think happens to a cow who can't produce milk anymore?" I asked.

"Well, I am sure the cow eventually dies, and then they probably bury her," she replied.

It would be nice to believe that dairy cows live to a ripe old age, die peacefully, and are buried by their caretakers, but the truth is, most dairy cows are destined, eventually, for the slaughterhouse.

Before you eat something, put it to the "**SOS**" test devised by Ingrid Newkirk. Ask yourself this question: "Was anyone **S**laughtered **O**r **S**tolen from to provide this food for me?" If the answer is "yes," then don't eat it.

Can we afford to care about the suffering of animals when so many human beings are starving? Yes, not only because caring about animals does not preclude caring about human beings, but because vegetarianism is of direct benefit to the planet and to reducing starvation around the world. A human child dies of malnutrition every two seconds on this planet, yet it takes fifteen to twenty pounds of grain to produce one pound of meat. If just ten percent of American meat eaters adopted a vegetarian diet, there would be twelve million more tons of grain to feed to humans—enough to support the sixty million people who starve to death each year.[26] When we come to understand the true benefits that come from the practice of asteya—nonstealing—the means to abolish human starvation will be realized, and all will have enough to eat.

---

[26] Rebecca Saltzberg, "The Steps to End World Hunger," Down to Earth <http://www.downtoearth.org/articles/end_hunger.htm>.

Chapter 5

BRAHMACHARYA

Good Sex

*At the Animal Research Institute, we are trying to breed
animals without legs and chickens without feathers.*
—R.S. GOWE, DIRECTOR OF THE ANIMAL RESEARCH INSTITUTE, AGRICULTURE
CANADA, SPEAKING AT AN AGRICULTURAL CONFERENCE IN OTTAWA[27]

Brahmacharya means "to respect the creative power of sex and
not abuse it by manipulating others sexually." What happens
when one becomes established in brahmacharya?

brahmacharya-pratishthayam virya-labhah PYS II.38
*When one does not misuse sexual energy, one obtains
enduring vitality resulting in good health.*

brahmacharya: not misusing sex (brahma: the creative
principle, god as creator + charya: vehicle or means to)
pratishthayam: being established or grounded in
virya: vigor, vitality
labhah: gained

---

[27] Jim Mason and Peter Singer, Animal Factories (New York: Harmony Books, 1990) 35.

BRAHMACHARYA IS A WAY TO GET TO GOD—A WAY TO ARRIVE AT THE creative essence of the universe. It has sometimes been translated as "continence" or "chastity," which I feel has led to a lot of misunderstanding in regard to how to practice this yama. To practice brahmacharya is to understand the potential of sexual energy, which is the essence of all physical and psychological forces. Sex is the power that creates life. When sexual energy is directed wisely, it becomes a means to transcend separation, or otherness. When sexual energy is used to exploit, manipulate, or humiliate another, however, it propels us into deeper separation and ignorance (avidya). Human beings routinely do this to the other species we confine in breeding facilities on farms. The sexual abuse of animals is ingrained in our culture, and it expresses itself in the practice of breeding, genetic manipulation, castration, artificial insemination, forced pregnancy, routine rape, and child abuse, which all fall under the category of "animal husbandry."

Animals on factory farms are not allowed to develop normal sexual relationships with others of their own species. Most confined animals never even see a member of the opposite sex of their own kind. All of the animals born in factory farms have come from mothers who have been artificially inseminated. These mothers will be repeatedly raped by human farmhands and forced to become pregnant over and over again until their fertility wanes, at which point they are slaughtered and eaten. Male animals chosen to be sperm donors are used and abused, live in constant frustration, and in the end are slaughtered as well. A male hog who is used as a sperm donor, for instance, is tethered and held in place while farm workers excite him by rubbing and massaging his testicles, penis, and foreskin until he is ready to ejaculate. The farm worker must then grab the animal's penis and aim it into a plastic "collection" pipe.

Such practices are violent, crass, and degrading to animals, and dehumanizing for the farm workers paid to do this work. The way these animals are routinely sexually abused reveals just how disconnected we have become from the natural world and the beauty and miracle of life.

Meat eating could be seen as a feminist issue; for if we believe in women's rights, we cannot condone and support the way female animals are exploited for milk, eggs, and babies. Most of the animals in our factory farms are female because they are the most exploitable, as they can provide milk as well as more babies. This has historically been the case in agriculture. Our culture is based on the exploitation of the feminine (Mother Nature), and so the eating of meat, eggs, and dairy products are an integral part of our system. If we feel that women should be treated fairly, then we must extend our desire for women's liberation to all women regardless of race, religion, *or species*. Yoga teaches us that what we do to others we ultimately do to ourselves. If we do not respect the rights of females of other species, how can we expect to successfully liberate human females?

Let's examine what happens to an average dairy cow on today's farms:

She lives in a tiny stall with a concrete floor in an indoor "milk facility" and has never seen the sun or stepped on ground or grass. She is not even a year old, yet she has just given birth to her first calf a few hours ago, which wasn't easy while being chained by the neck. She had tried to lie down, but it was hard, and harder to get back up. Now the tethering chain makes it difficult for her to get close to her baby, but the baby is there, she knows. The baby is nursing, but not for long. Within hours, men come to take her baby. They shout at her, using harsh words. She tries to turn her head to see what is happening, but the chain prevents her from moving. She cries out to her baby, who cries back. In a few minutes, she no longer hears the cries of her newborn. He is in a truck being driven to a "veal facility," and his cries are out of her range of hearing. She is left in her place, her milk dripping from her breasts.

The milking machine now mechanically moves into place and clamps onto her nipples, sucking her and emptying her of the vital life force, which was intended for her baby. The machine will come again two more times today and most every day after that. She is crying and desperate to know what has happened to her baby. She becomes sad and depressed for weeks.

Soon after, a farm worker returns to her stall. She is chained, unable to turn around, defenseless when he inseminates her. She has given birth, had her baby stolen from her, been milked excessively by a machine, and now she is being raped. The worker first inserts his hand, then forces his arm up to his elbow into her vagina to open it up and locate her uterus. He then lodges the inseminator, a long, stainless-steel syringe, into her vagina and pumps sperm into her to impregnate her. She is now lactating and pregnant. She has to be pregnant or lactating to be able to produce milk, and in our culture, producing milk is the reason for her existence. She is viewed as a milk machine, a slave, one of billions of cows confined in factory-farm concentration camps.

In 1940, the average milk cow in the United States produced two tons of milk per year. Today a dairy cow, thanks to artificial insemination, genetic engineering, antibiotics, growth hormones, and cheap "enriched" feed, produces up to ten tons per year. To get a cow to produce that much milk is unnatural and requires drastic measures. A cow by nature is vegan, eating only plant foods, so to be able to produce the amount of milk that will turn a profit, she is force-fed the flesh of other animals. It is common practice on today's farms to feed chickens, turkeys, cows, pigs, sheep, and goats "enriched" feed. Enriched feed is made of genetically modified corn, soy, oats, or wheat and laced with the rendered remains of slaughtered animals. Rendered meat by-products contain not only the body parts of animals raised in factory farms (chickens, turkeys, pigs, sheep, goats, and cows) but also dead animals collected from laboratories, zoos, schools, city shelters, circuses, puppy and kitten mills; road kill; and fish. Most of the fish caught by commercial trawlers is not eaten by humans but fed to livestock. The FDA assures us that since the outbreaks of bovine spongiform encephalopathy (BSE, or "mad cow" disease), the "enriched" feed that is fed to cows doesn't include other cows in the recipe; nevertheless it still includes their brains and spinal cords.[28]

Once pregnant again, the dairy cow remains chained by the neck in her stall with nothing to do but stand on concrete day in and day out, enduring the milking machine that empties her several times a day, until the last two months of her pregnancy, when she won't be milked. Even though she just stands there, her body is working very hard to produce all that milk and carry a baby in her womb. The amount of energy she expends is equivalent to what a human would if he were to jog for six hours every day.[29] But this cow isn't able to get any exercise, as she can't move, and her udders become so full that they drag on the concrete floor and are heavy, swollen, and painful. The milking machine cuts her sometimes and causes sores; at other times, it gives her an electric shock, which makes her continuously afraid and anxious.

She is impregnated every year until she is four years old. By that time, she is physically and emotionally broken and her milk production is waning, so she is scheduled to be taken off the milking machine.

Farm workers arrive, and for the first time in her life, they unchain her from her stall. They push her roughly, trying to get

---

[28] Dave Syerson, "Questions and Answers Concerning Pet Food Regulations," Association of American Feed Control Officials, Inc. 18 Aug. 2008 <http://www.aafco.org>.

[28] David C. Coats, Old MacDonald's Factory Farm (New York: Continuum, 1989) 55.

her out of her stall. She is afraid and confused, and her legs are sore. The men are forcing her to walk. She has never walked before and doesn't know what is expected of her. The workers push and shove her and prod her with a device that gives her an electric shock. Somehow she manages to get out of the building. This is also happening to many of the other cows who have been in the building with her for the last four years. They are all loaded into a large truck. It is very crowded in the truck, and all of them are afraid. They peer through the slats in the sides of the truck. They have never seen the light of day; they have never seen anything except the inside of their stall in the milking facility. It is cold, and their udders are full of milk and very sore. They travel for a long time, as it becomes dark and then light again. The truck stops, and when the door opens the men pull and push them out of the truck. The cows hear screaming and smell blood; they become terrified. The more scared they become, the more violent and impatient the men are, yanking and kicking them to move them faster. Some of the cows collapse, their legs just giving out on them. The men kick and use electric prods to shock these downed cows into standing up and walking. If that doesn't work, they may use a hose to force water up their noses to try to get them to stand and walk into the slaughterhouse.

The cow somehow makes it into the new building, but she senses that it is a place of death. She can't escape, and as before, she is unable to turn around. As a worker tries to shoot a steel pellet into her head, she moves, and instead, he shoots her in her left eye. She is shackled and yanked up into the air, her heavy body hanging from one leg. She is seeing so much suffering and death. She is crying, but no one seems to be listening. A man with a large sharp—or worse, dull—knife cuts her throat, shoves his hand into this cruel wound, and pulls out her trachea. She struggles to get free. She is conscious and aware, but there is no one to help her. She hangs upside down bleeding to death. Next some other men begin to cut and dismember her body. As they cut into her abdomen, the baby she has been carrying in her womb falls out onto the killing floor.

Her body, once viewed as a milking machine, is now just so much meat and will most likely end up as cheap hamburger in a fast-food restaurant. The baby she was carrying? Its body will be skinned, and the soft leather will be sold as expensive calfskin.

As many former workers have verified, the animal-user industries consider abuse normal in factory farms and slaughterhouses. There are many incidences of slaughterhouse workers being caught on undercover film sexually abusing the animals whom they are also killing and dismembering. There are also incidences of farm workers sexually abusing confined and tethered animals in factory farms. As most animals are tethered (held in place by ropes, chains, or straps), they are acutely vulnerable to abuse. Many female pigs are strapped down to a concrete floor, unable to move. Veal calves, having been taken away from their mothers at birth and confined in small crates, are desperate to suck and will suck on anything. Some farm workers take advantage of these disadvantaged baby animals. These are not a few isolated incidences—it is widespread.[30] The only difference between sexually abusing an animal in a slaughterhouse and raping an animal confined in a factory farm is that what happens to the animal in the factory farm is commonly accepted and excused as part of the necessary business of breeding, and what goes on in the slaughterhouses is considered "not procedure." Either way the same thing is going on—an animal is being brutally and intimately violated without his or her consent.

Is there any reason to doubt the connection between widespread pornography and this kind of unspeakable

---

[30] Visit **www.peta.org** or **www.hsus.org** to see acts like these caught on film.

animal exploitation? Both are rooted in the blind ambition to dominate—the antithesis of a yogi's instinct and pursuit. Both are considered acceptable, tolerated, and possibly even "normal" within our culture, one that is based on the degradation of the feminine and disconnection from the sacredness of life.

Consider the snuff film—the epitome of perverse pornography. The finale is the murder of a woman, preferably pregnant, her abdomen sliced open and her uterus cut out. Pornography is just a symptom of a culture in which the subjugation, rape, and dismembering of animals occurs all day, every day. When you watch undercover films of workers on factory farms or in slaughterhouses, you hear over and over again the workers roughly and angrily shouting at the terrified animals, calling them names that reference and degrade female sexuality: "bitch," "cunt," "whore," etc.

The parallels to the relationship between the sexes are undeniable. Some men frequently refer to women as "pussy," "bunny," "cow," "pig," and "chick," and to their body parts as choice cuts of meat: large hams and pieces of ass. A man may voice his preference in women by saying, "I'm a breast man" or, "I'm a thigh man." Of course the stereotypical female sex symbol, like the domesticated cow, turkey, or chicken, has to have excessively large breasts.

There is no doubt in my mind that the wearing of high heels by women is definitely a cultural aberration—symbolic of a culture accustomed to dismembering animals and hanging their parts in the butcher's window. When naked and walking on high heels, a human female, viewed from behind, bears a striking resemblance to the hindquarters of a cow, goat, or pig—animals whose hooves have the effect of elevating their rumps, making them look like they are walking on tiptoes. Advertisements for rib joints or barbecue restaurants often use images of pigs and cows wearing high heels and skimpy clothes.

The consumption of meat and dairy products, like the use of pornography which degrades women, is a symptom of the disease of low self-esteem. Both activities result from the misguided notion that in order to feel sexier, younger, healthier, or stronger, one must exploit and consume the gifts of nature in any form that man can readily dominate. In fact, the opposite is true. Long-term consumption of meat and dairy products can create any number of health problems, including heart disease, impotence, stroke, and cancer.

There is a higher incidence of impotence among meat eaters than vegetarians. A diet high in cholesterol is linked to sexual disorders.[31] The huge rise in the sales of pharmaceutical drugs used to increase sexual potency is evidence of our meat-eating culture's fear of losing virility. In India, milk drinking was, and still is, equated with male virility and the abundance of healthy sperm, but research has shown that drinking milk can clog the arteries and therefore increase a man's chances of developing erectile dysfunction.[32]

In modern times, eating meat and dairy products has been strongly linked to disease—not to health. Many diseases that have plagued human beings over the centuries stem from our mistreatment of animals. The stress of confinement suffered by enslaved animals brought about certain pathologies. With time, mutations allowed diseases to jump species: trichinosis and tuberculosis were originally diseases found in domesticated pigs; human influenza came from avian flu; horsepox mutated into smallpox; bovine rinderpest became measles;[33] and variant Creutzfeldt-Jakob disease is the human equivalent of mad cow disease.

In *The World Without Us*, Alan Weisman asks, "Could AIDS be the animals' final revenge? The human immunode-

---

[31] Maria Esposito, "Is High Cholesterol Harming Your Sex Life," Fox News 13 Aug. 2008 <http://www.foxnews.com/story/0,2933,403384,00.html>.

[32] "Impotence," Go Veg <http://www.goveg.com/impotence.asp>.

[33] Charles C. Mann, 1491: New Revelations of the Americas Before Columbus (New York: Alfred A. Knopf, 2006) 98-99.

ficiency virus that infects people is closely related to a simian strain that chimps carry without getting sick. Infection probably spread to humans through bush meat. On encountering the 4 percent of our genes that differ from the genes of our closest primate relations, the virus mutated lethally."[34]

Patanjali tells us very clearly that health and vitality will come to one who is established in brahmacharya; to one who treats sexuality with reverence. If we want to be healthy, we must consider the suffering, disease, and ill health we are causing to the animals we eat. Can we really expect to be healthy by causing so much disease in the lives of others?

To embrace the practice of brahmacharya is to challenge our culture's foundation, which is dependent upon the domestication of animals. When we talk about veganism and the practice of brahmacharya, we are definitely talking about a radical sexual revolution.

---

[34] Alan Weisman, The World Without Us (New York: Thomas Dunne Books, 2007) 86.

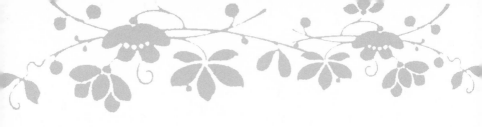

Chapter 6

APARIGRAHA

Greed, Excess, and Poverty

---

*Whatever joy there is in this world all comes from desiring
others to be happy, and whatever suffering there is in this
world all comes from desiring myself to be happy.*
—Shantideva, *A Guide to the Bodhisattva Way of Life*

Aparigraha means "greedlessness." What happens when one
becomes established in greedlessness?

aparigraha-sthairye janma-kathamta-sambodhah PYS II.39
*When one becomes selfless and ceases to take more than one
needs, one obtains knowledge of why one was born.*

aparigraha: greedlessness (**a:** not + **pari:** toward + **graha:** grasp)
sthairye: being settled or established in
janma: birth
kathamta: process of why and how
sambodhah: one has knowledge

WHEN WE DESIRE HAPPINESS FOR OURSELVES AT THE EXPENSE OF
others, it is called "greed." Patanjali recommends that yogis
seeking enlightenment should try to live a simple life based
in moderation rather than excessive consumption. In other

words, "Live simply so that others may simply live." This is a radical concept to embrace these days, but yogis have always been radical.

Patanjali says that those who become established in aparigraha will come to know their future, as they obtain knowledge of the processes that resulted in their birth. This is because the practitioner comes to a deep understanding that his birth, life, imminent physical death, and the entire world he is experiencing is being created from his actions. The yogi begins to understand emptiness (*shunyata*)—how actions arise from one's perception of reality and how reality is never separate from one's perception of it. The yogi expands his perception of reality beyond the confines of linear time, dropping into a heightened state of awareness, which is the eternity of the present moment. This heightened state of awareness enables one to live more fully and more feelingly. As sensuality develops, empathy follows, lifting one out of self-centeredness into other-centeredness.

Through the practice of greedlessness, a yogi transcends linear time and is able to be free of wants. When we begin to contemplate the potential infinite results of our actions, we may begin to reflect on whether or not we can karmically afford certain actions.

Real needs are not wrong; wants, on the other hand, can become problematic. We are in the midst of a global crisis caused by insatiable human greed. The more we have, the more we want. Influenced by media imagery and advertising, we have become habituated to look outside of ourselves for happiness and, in the process, have created powerful addictions that drive our choices. Each time we allow an outside stimulus to program our actions, we allow our own inner power of discrimination to atrophy a bit, leading to further addiction. Many of us have become so out of touch with our innermost selves that we do not know where need ends and want begins. We become confused and use phrases like, "I need to buy a new car" or, "The kids need new school clothes" or, "I really need you to do this for me" or, "I need a drink," as if we would die without it. We identify with what we have, need, and want. Due to *avidya* (ignorance), which gives rise to *asmita* (excessive identification with ego), we think we are our personalities, and with that thinking we lose touch with the true Self. The Self, which is whole and complete in its interconnectedness with all of existence, is sustained by love. One who identifies with this Self is a holy being, who knows when enough is enough and will never jeopardize the existence of the whole society for his or her wants.

A yogi practices self-reflection. This gives rise to *viveka* (discrimination), out of which arises wisdom, which leads to making choices that lead to enlightenment—not into deeper ignorance.

We have consumed far more than we need. The consequences for the survival of many animal species, as well as our own, are dire. The directive aparigraha, in contrast, helps one curb one's actions in accordance with what is good for all. Through aparigraha, we begin to understand ourselves as holy beings who thrive as part of a whole organism, working together for common benefit. We begin to feel our unique contribution to the wholeness of life. We come to understand that what we do is not small or insignificant to the lives of others or to the planet, but reverberates through every living being through time and space eternally. We become truly Self-conscious as we begin to realize ourselves as part of the greater whole of life and understand our destiny.

It is often argued that we alone possess consciousness and that all other animals do not and are only acting from an instinctual awareness, implying that they don't know why they are doing something or how their actions might affect themselves or others. For this reason, many people think that animals are a lower life form and are less conscious and therefore undeserving of the same considerations we might extend to other human beings. I believe that animals are conscious. But, like us, some are more conscious of themselves and the world around them, and some are less so, and this can be influenced by age and illness. *Consciousness* means "joint mutual knowledge." The Oxford English Dictionary breaks the word down into: *con*=with, together + *science*=knowing of the whole. Thus the word *self-consciousness* means "knowledge of one's self as connected to the whole."

I have contemplated the assumption that animals are not conscious for many years while watching the way the deer and wild birds come to eat in our backyard in upstate New York. Never have I seen a deer or bird remain and eat all the food before moving on. A deer will come and take a few mouthfuls of grass, leaves, or seeds, lift her head and chew slowly, maybe lower her head and take another mouthful and repeat, and then walk away, allowing the next passing deer to sample some of the remaining food. I have never observed any wild animal staying and eating until there was no more food left. Nor have I ever seen any wild animal come with a bag or backpack, shovel in the food, fill the bag, and then carry it away so that there would be nothing left for others. No other animal besides us would destroy a whole forest or cause the extinction of entire species while imagining that it has no negative effect upon them or the lives of their future children.

Some people say that animals are less intelligent than we are because they don't make stuff. They don't build houses or shopping malls; print newspapers or magazines; manufacture rockets, airplanes, cars, or boats; or make plastic bags, televisions, VCRs, cell phones, or computers. Perhaps animals have more developed intelligence and greater consciousness than we do, when measured by the ability to make connections. Many animals, because of their greedlessness, seem to have a deeper sense of how their actions might affect the greater whole. As they have managed to live without destroying their habitats, unlike us, perhaps many of the other animals are more conscious than we are.

If greedlessness leads to awareness, greed leads to denial. Many of us receive our first lesson in denial as children, when we question the morality of eating meat. As previously mentioned in the Prologue, when I was a child, I asked my mother, "If killing is wrong, isn't it wrong to eat animals?" My mother replied, "It's okay because they are raised for that." This confused me even more. Another common response to that moral question is, "Yes, it is wrong, but it is a necessary evil." In his book *Dominion*, Matthew Scully responds with the question, "When is evil ever *really necessary?*"

The Oxford English Dictionary provides the Germanic *ubel* as the root word for *evil*. Ubel means "up" or "over," meaning to go beyond the limits of what is proper. In other words, that which is excessive is evil.

Earth provides enough to satisfy every man's need, but not every man's greed.
—Mahatma Gandhi

According to the United Nations Food and Agriculture Organization, over fifty-two billion animals are killed for food worldwide every year.[35] If you visit the website: **www.abolistionistapproach.com,** you can see the number of individual animals killed in the world every second. In the United States alone, approximately ten billion land animals and billions of sea creatures are slaughtered for food each year. It is hard to know how many sea creatures are killed because they are not counted as individuals but by tonnage. Regardless, anyway

[35] Visit the Food and Agriculture Organization of the United Nations' Global Livestock Production and Health Atlas (GLiPHA) at **www.fao.org** as well as "Worldwide Animal Slaughter Statistics (based on FAO numbers)" at **www.sfvegan.org**.

you look at it, these are staggering numbers, especially if you consider that the human population of the United States is around three hundred and four million, and that there are over six billion human beings on the entire planet. These billions of suffering and terrified animals create a planetary atmosphere of fear, terror, and violence, which we all live and breathe in everyday. One could easily call this amount of animal slaughter excessive. Farley Mowat writes in the book *Sea of Slaughter*: "The living world is dying in our time…. When our forebears commenced their exploitation of this continent they believed the animate resources of the New World were infinite and inexhaustible. The vulnerability of that living fabric—the intricacy and fragility of its all too finite parts—was beyond their comprehension. It can…be said in their defense that they were mostly ignorant of the inevitable consequences of their dreadful depredations. We who are alive today can claim no such exculpation for our biocidal actions and their dire consequences."[36]

We are devastating our oceans and emptying them of life. Many sea creatures are now extinct, and the number of threatened species is growing. Captain Paul Watson, founder of the Sea Shepherd Conservation Society, says, "Seafood is simply a socially acceptable form of bush meat. We condemn Africans for hunting monkeys and mammalian and bird species from the jungle, yet the developed world thinks nothing of hauling in magnificent wild creatures like swordfish, tuna, halibut, shark and salmon for our meals. The fact is that the global slaughter of marine life is simply the largest massacre of wildlife on the planet."[37]

Human beings do not eat all of the fish that is caught; most of it is force-fed to confined animals in factory farms to fatten them for slaughter. It may take twelve pounds of grain to make one pound of hamburger, but it also takes a hundred pounds of fish to make that one pound of hamburger.[38] Force-feeding

---

[36] Farley Mowat, Sea of Slaughter (Mechanicsburg, PA: Stackpole Books, 2004) 383.
[37] "The Veg News Interview: Captain Paul Watson." Veg News March-April 2003: 25.
[38] Ibid, 27.

animals, like cows who by nature are herbivores (vegetarians), the flesh of other animals—and sometimes even of their own species—could be deemed excessive and therefore evil.

Sea creatures suffer in other ways due to human greed. They starve to death because of lack of food. Their world is polluted by the toxic chemicals that we continuously flush into the ocean. Large fishing trawlers rake up many sea creatures that they did not intend to catch. The fishing industry refers to these beings as "by-catch." When the hauls are sorted out, most of these creatures are either dead or dying and cannot survive the trauma of being caught. They are thrown back into the ocean like so much garbage.

The relationship of humans to the Earth and all its creatures has been largely opportunistic, exploitative, and violent. It has resulted in a system of subjugation, domination, and exploitation. We see the results of this all around us in the world today: pollution, slavery, war, division, nationalism, sexism, speciesism, and extinction. There is an alternative: live so that your own life enhances, rather than impoverishes, the lives of others. This is not a new message. It is an ancient message with new-found meaning for the crisis we face today.

In my worldwide travels teaching yoga, I have found that human beings are pretty much the same all over; we are all looking for happiness. For the most part, the people I meet who are interested in yoga are dissatisfied with the present culture, which propagates the idea that happiness can only be achieved through material wealth gained through the exploitation of the Earth and other beings. The people I meet seem to want to break free from a commodity-driven way of life to find a new way of living that is more kind, simple, fulfilling, and selfless.

As His Holiness the Dalai Lama recommends, "Think of the problems in the whole world as your fault." To care for others is in our own self-interest. His Holiness calls this "enlightened self-interest." To dare to care about the happiness of others is to awaken the power of unconditional love within you.

te samadhav upasarga vyutthane siddhayah PYS III.38
By giving up the love of power, you attain the power of love.

te: they (referring to the *siddhis* or powers)
samadhav: for the attainment of enlightenment; cosmic love
upasarga: obstacle
vyutthane: outward show
siddhayah: supernatural powers

Jimi Hendrix must have been channeling this yoga sutra. In any case, the message of love as the greatest power continues to ring true. The power of love cures the disease of low self-esteem, which is a pandemic in our world today. There are no "ordinary people!" Everyone is a manifestation of the Divine. Through the practice of yoga, people begin to remember this. They become Self-confident through a deep inner connection with the eternal Self, which is the real essence of every being. The nature of that inner Self is joy.

When one feels this joy and confidence, one is less likely to hurt others. The underlying reason that we hurt others is our ignorance (*avidya*): we don't see the soul and divinity in other forms of life. This is at the core of the question of why human beings eat meat, enslave and exploit animals, and go to war with other people. If we felt Self-confident, we would not be inclined toward violence and greed. We would have a peaceful world free of poverty, slavery, and war.

Through the practices of yoga, we discover that concern for the happiness and well-being of others, including other animals, must be an essential part of our own quest for happiness and well-being. We realize that we can never be free as long as we participate in enslaving others. As our ability to be compassionate and extend our compassion to include animals grows, we heal the disease of disconnection so prevalent in our culture, and we begin to feel whole again.

We begin to see that it could be possible to create peace on Earth while living a liberated life—the life of the jivanmukta. Through adopting a compassionate, vegetarian way of eating, we take the first big step toward becoming established in aparigraha, and with that, we step into a bright, enlightened future for ourselves, for the animals, and for this planet.

Our culture has conditioned us over thousands of years to hoard, stockpile, accumulate, and save for a rainy day. The amount of things we feel we own gives us a sense of security and creates a legacy of self-importance that we want to pass on to our children in the hopes of being remembered or immortalized. Buying power is a much sought after *siddhi* in our modern times.

Shopping is a major part of most human lives. Much of what we work so hard to buy we don't even really want. Soon we get tired of it and throw it away, thus creating "throw away" or "disposable" societies. I read that eight-five percent of everything purchased in an American shopping mall ends up in a landfill within two weeks after purchase. The activist Julia Butterfly Hill asks, "Where is this place we call 'away?'" Of course, it doesn't exist. Each time we designate something as trash, we lose something of our own souls in the process. In the languages of many indigenous cultures, where there is perhaps more of a kinship felt with other animals and the Earth, there are no words for trash or garbage; the concept of throwing something away doesn't even exist.

Our consuming and hoarding behavior has been evolving for thousands of years. Early on, when we began to domesticate and enslave animals and to farm the land, we also developed methods to preserve the surplus of harvested food.

We came to think of the flesh and milk of animals in the same way as the vegetables we plant, grow, harvest, and hoard—as wealth that enables us to market, buy, and sell. Over thousands of years, we have cultivated this way of life and the belief in the necessity of it. We instill in our children a certainty about the need to work and along with it the concept that work somehow differs from life itself.

We divide our lives into workdays and vacations, or days off. Many of us think of work as something we do to enable us to live, but do not consider it something that we like or prefer doing. This is a strange idea, since during the many hours that we spend working, we are also alive! Still, we often feel that our work is not what we really want to be doing, that it is only a means to an end, and that our real life begins after work.

We have created a relationship with time in which we believe that life is made up of a series of events, the causes of which are random, and the end result a mystery. Civilized humans have lost their connection with the cycles of nature. We have become time-bound, enslaved to the clock and wristwatch. When we exist fully in the present moment, there is less fear of not having enough in the future and less inclination to greedily stockpile a surplus. Through the practice of aparigraha, the yogi becomes conscious of his or her true existence as having never been born and with that realization is able to defeat death. For it is only those who insist they were born who will die.

Yoga provides a door to the infinite through the experience of multi-dimensional reality. Eternity is happening now for the yogi who becomes unfettered by the conventional restraints of linear time. Such a yogi dismantles the ancient prison walls built by the bricks of greed and held together by the mortar of fear. All fears come down to the fear of losing: losing fame, youth, money, hair, health, love...but ultimately life. If one thinks of himself as mortal, his whole life will be haunted by the fear of death (*abhinivesha*) which, according to Patanjali, is a great hindrance to Yoga. To let go of the desire to possess is to be liberated from the fear of death.

When the yogi realizes the eternity of the Self, he becomes unbound by time and freed from the cycle of birth, life, and death. This new level of consciousness allows the imagination to explore the infinite possibilities of simultaneous existences. As one becomes unchained from linearity, the illusion of rational thought dissolves as intuition dawns. This dawning will be swift and timely as intuition envelops the parts into the whole to give birth to a brand new day.

We are on the brink of an apocalypse that some have prophesied will result in a radical shift in how we relate to time. The Greek word *apocalypse* means "to reveal; to uncover; to stand naked, exposed without artifice, clothing, or possessions." When we let go of holding on to things, our hands will be open to receive everything.

This present age, or *yuga*, has been spoken of in Hindu scripture as the *Kali Yuga*. *Kali* is derived from the Sanskrit word *kala*, meaning "time." Some say that in the year 2012, perhaps there will be an end to time as we have come to know it. It will be the end of a long-standing relationship with time as distinct from the infinite aspect of space, and with it will come a glorious revelation of new possibilities. A new age will be born. As with all births, it will be a bloody matter, but it will result in wondrous potential. Perhaps our true potential will be revealed to us as caring, nurturing beings who see ourselves as an essential part of a whole—who see ourselves as holy.

Certainly, we must all agree that our present greed-driven, consumer-based culture will not sustain the Earth or us, as it is destined to throw us all away. We must find a more harmonious and mutually beneficial way to live with all beings, where we distinguish between need and greed and act accordingly. Technological advancements are happening at an accelerating pace, but is our consciousness? Until we actually feel infinity, time will run out, and we will never experience a time/space continuum: a multi-dimensional place not bound by the past or future. It won't be too long now until time will be no longer, and death will be the last thing to die.

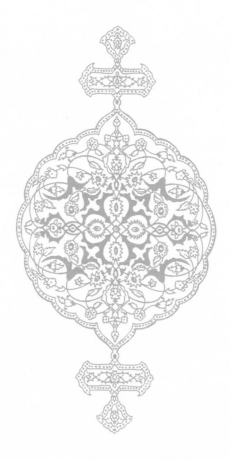

Chapter 7

LIVING THE LIFE OF A JIVANMUXTA

Spiritual Activism

Never doubt that a small group of thoughtful committed citizens can change the world. Indeed, it is the only thing that ever has.
—Margaret Mead

JIVA MEANS "INDIVIDUAL SOUL" AND *MUXTA* MEANS "LIBERATION." A *jivanmukta* is a liberated soul—one who knows him- or herself to be one with all that is. A jivanmukta is a living liberated being who works to contribute to the liberation of others.

An activist is someone who actively works for change. To be spiritual is to feel your connection to all living beings. Spiritual activism is to actively work to further the conscious connection of oneself to others in a positive, life-affirming, mutually beneficial way. To be a spiritual activist is to be activated by spirit rather than a skin-encapsulated ego. To dare to care about the happiness, well-being, and liberation of others is to be a spiritual activist. A jivanmukta actively pursues liberation or enlightenment for the benefit of all.

The biggest obstacle to our spiritual evolution as a species at this time is our perception and treatment of animals and the natural world. Once we wake up from our sleep of denial and become aware of the truth of our connection to all of life, our spiritual practice, or *sadhana*, begins.

Philosopher Arthur Schopenhauer said, "All truth passes through three stages. First, it is ridiculed. Second, it is violently opposed. Third, it is accepted as being self-evident." After you are exposed to the truth of how animals are treated by today's agribusiness and how the members of our worldwide culture perpetuate this treatment through the meals they eat and products they buy, it will be difficult for you to continue to live the life you previously led. The most difficult thing for many people who become awakened to the reality of animal abuse is to figure out how they are going to help stop the abuse. Inaction is not an option for the yogi, but how to act in the most effective way may not be so obvious, at first.

When people learn of the horrible animal abuse that goes on day after day, they typically react in one of two ways. Either they feel despairing, overwhelmed, and helpless, or they get angry and want to attack the perpetrators.

Neither one of these reactions will bring about a positive transformation that will benefit the animals. It will take intense passion of the best type: compassion. Only through active, conscious compassion can you affect people's minds and hearts, with the result that they find it in themselves to be compassionate and to extend that compassion to all beings, including animals. In other words, change must start with you; you must become the embodiment of compassion. You must treat the people you are speaking with in a compassionate manner no matter how outraged you may feel. Even though you now know the facts about how animals are abused and how this is causing mass destruction of the planet as well as our spirits and our health, you must use yogic self-control and temper your passion with compassion. If you come across as preachy, angry, or judgmental, you most likely will not be able to hold an audience long enough for them to begin to hear the truth of what you are saying.

As you begin to speak of the truth you have experienced about how animals are treated, you will likely be ridiculed by others at first, even by friends and family members. Accept this as a natural phase in the process for people whose lifelong conditioned assumptions are being challenged. Hang in there, and stick with your principles. Patanjali suggests that when you find yourself in a difficult situation, turn it upside down. See it as an opportunity, not as an obstacle, and, most importantly, don't get angry.

vitarka-badhane pratipaksha-bhavanam PYS II.33
When disturbed by disturbing thoughts, think of the opposite.

vitarka: negative thought
badhane: to overcome; make beneficial
pratipaksha: the opposite
bhavanam: should be thought of

When destructive emotions like hate, anger, or the desire to do violence arise within you, cultivate the opposite state of mind. See the other person's potential for kindness and bolster your own expression of kindness. View others with hope, seeing them as having overcome their own ignorance. If you see them in a negative way, the power of your perception will only help to keep them that way as you polarize yourself from them, assuming a superior role.

The ridicule you may endure from others when you speak up for animals can help you to hone your skills, enabling you to become better at articulating the message of veganism and animal rights in an informed and compassionate way.

As the others around you realize that your principles will not be easily shaken by their dismissive attitude, they may come to feel threatened. When people's lifelong habits and assumptions are threatened, they may display violent opposition to the truths you are helping them to realize. When huge corporations feel financial threats to their profits, they will undoubtedly react with aggressive opposition. Remember: the key to the success of the animal-user industries has been the ignorance of the consumers and their unquestioned trust in authority. As the stakes get higher, the animal-user industries and their long-standing governmental supporters will take drastic measures against those who act to support the liberation of animals from human exploitation. Hang in there. This is only phase two. Acceptance of truth is bound to come, because it is what underlies our ground of being. The truth is that we are one, appearing as many. How we treat each other will be reflected in the individual, as well as in the whole. Many people, when they finally come to accept something as truth, will deny that they were ever in opposition to it. Fine; don't worry about that. Celebrate every step anyone takes toward becoming more conscious and more whole. The steps to truth are the steps to holiness.

> *The individual is capable of both great compassion and great indifference. Humans have it within their means to nourish the former and outgrow the latter. Nothing is more powerful than an individual acting out of conscience, thus helping to bring the collective consciousness to life.*
> —NORMAN COUSINS, JOURNALIST AND PEACE ACTIVIST

Now that you have an understanding of the yamas and how the way that you treat others not only affects them, but also affects what happens to you, you will be able to go beyond an intellectual grasp of the concepts provided by Patanjali and experiment through experience and reflection. You will experience proof of these ideas through the daily experiences provided by your own life.

Others will undoubtedly ask you questions like how and why you practice yoga, and why you eat the way you do. I hope the following advice will help you connect to that innate, compassionate part of yourself where your unique problem-solving skills lie, waiting to be expressed.

The real question is how to unearth and develop compassion within yourself so that it is what motivates your interactions with others. Compassion is the essential tool if you want to be an effective speaker on the subject of yoga and vegetarianism. If you have a desire to speak to people and help them understand why they should care about animals and adopt a vegetarian diet, then these ideas may help you achieve your goals.

I. LISTENING: The *Heart* of Communication

FIRST, BE SURE YOU *WANT* TO COMMUNICATE. MANY PEOPLE ARE ONLY concerned with expressing themselves, which isn't necessarily communication. Communication implies communing, having a shared experience with another, not "talking at" someone. Merely professing what you know is not communicating. Listening is essential to communication, taking into consideration the person you are talking to and where he or she may be coming from. Through empathy, consider why people might be doing certain things that you would like them to change. To develop empathy toward someone who is doing something you consider morally or ethically wrong, try to realize these facts:

1. Whenever people are doing anything, they are doing the best they can at that time.

2. When someone is doing something abusive, they are getting something that they feel is positive from the experience.

Through empathetic listening, you will be able to change underlying causes, not just outward symptoms. Nonviolent communication with others whom you would like to inspire toward change will transform you in the process, as it will develop compassion, which dissolves differences and leads to an enlightened existence.

If we, as yoga teachers and practitioners, are to communicate the radical ideas of yoga, we must address controversial topics such as animal rights and vegetarianism. To do so successfully, we must focus our time, efforts, and skills to their greatest effect. It will serve no one if we get burned out, losing sleep over the fact that we haven't accomplished world peace, the end of war, and global veganism overnight. Instead, we can make real gains by focusing on specific real opportunities that surround us every day, such as the people who come through our doors seeking yoga, those who are asking us to teach them the means to become happy.

A yoga teacher is a communicator, not a professor. To communicate, one must be able to listen and to hear where the other is coming from. A yoga teacher must begin with an understanding of compassion as the ultimate cause of enlightenment. Whatever methods the teacher shares with the student should awaken compassion within the student—compassion not only for others, but for themselves as well.

When we want to speak about yoga to someone who is still eating meat and does not see the karmic connections between what they are doing and their present physical, emotional, mental, or spiritual condition—or even their potential future condition—we must first find a way to communicate with them. It's no use condemning them. Instead we must listen in order to "hear" their present condition.

Eating meat and consuming milk products is an addiction: an addiction to violence. To facilitate a lasting positive change, we must view the person who is still eating these foods in the same light as we would view a drug or a sex addict.

Rational arguments usually don't have much effect on addicts. Drug addicts, for example, may have an intellectual understanding of their problem, and may even say they want to stop, but they can't because of physiological and psychological addiction. A better approach to the issue would be to appeal to the heart of the addict. This takes skillful communication, starting with the ability to listen. One must be careful not to condemn violent acts through guilt. Guilt is not an effective way to initiate a lasting change of heart in an addict. We must go to the heart and help the person enter into a deeper feeling level of his or her own being and connection with all other beings. This is what a yoga teacher does.

We must probe deeper and try to understand the possible motives for the person's actions. When someone is engaged in a "bad" action, in their mind they believe that they are getting something "good" from the action. If we want to try to help someone stop destructive actions, we have to look at the benefit the person thinks he or she is getting. We must view the person through the eyes of compassion. We must see them as whole and complete and communicate to them from that viewpoint, recognizing that their habit of causing harm to others is coming from a deep feeling of incompleteness within themselves. We must address the *avidya*, or underlying lack of true Self-confidence and of Self-esteem. To begin to do so, we must first find a way to communicate, which means listening to the suffering of that other person; this will awaken our compassion and provide us with the skills to take the necessary actions. We must discover the cause of their actions, not merely address or condemn the symptoms.

I recall an interview with psychologist Marshall Rosenberg, in which he described his work with prisoners incarcerated for being child molesters. Dr. Rosenberg spoke about one particular prisoner who had shared his story after several sessions. As with many cases of child abuse, the prisoner himself had been abused as a child. When asked by the doctor to describe his childhood experience, the prisoner vividly described the horror and trauma he had gone through at that time. He also intimated that his experience had been all the more horrific because he could not communicate his fear and terror to anyone. Even when he had tried to communicate, he found that the other person could not understand what he was describing because they had not been there and felt what he had felt. Dr. Rosenberg then asked the obvious question, "If it was such a horrific experience for you, then why would you want to do this to other children?" The prisoner replied, "When I saw the fear and terror in the child's face, I knew, at last, that I was with someone who understood what I had gone through."[39]

Perhaps all of the violence in the world today could be seen in essence as a failed attempt to communicate. True communication depends upon not just one party expressing themselves, but both parties listening to each other and developing a shared expression.

Through compassion, real communication is possible. If we, as activists, want to stop violence against animals, we must offer a clear, lasting, positive solution that will satisfy all parties. We can't just condemn and vent anger against meat eaters. This is an important point for the activist to remember. We must override the tendency within ourselves to perpetuate the good guys/bad guys, winner/loser, or victim/perpetrator syndrome.

---

[39] Marshall Rosenberg, Speaking Peace: Connecting With Others Through Non-Violent Communication, Sounds True, 2003.

Our ultimate aim must be a win-win outcome for all: for the animals, the former animal exploiter, and even ourselves.

Yoga provides practical methods to communicate through developing one's ability to listen. Take, for instance, the yogic method of practicing asanas—especially twisting asanas. They address on a gut level the ego or separate-self and bring awareness to the organs of digestion and assimilation of food. This can awaken latent or buried feelings of anger, depression, or low self-esteem, which have been subtly held in those organs. Through practicing asanas, one can begin to unearth the causes of their destructive tendencies and heal the disconnection. People eat meat in an attempt to feel better about themselves—to feel healthier, sexier, stronger, or more empowered. They mistakenly feel that by taking the life of another, they will gain power. Instead, they become addicted to an illusion of power and are ultimately weakened, because their sense of power comes from disempowering another, not from the source of power itself, the Self, which resides within and whose nature is unconditional love. This ignorance or mis-knowing is a case of mistaken identity and leads to deeper external and internal disconnection and further violence. And as the process is repeated over and over again, the person finds him- or herself caught in a net of debilitating addiction. The yoga student, through the practice of twisting asanas, becomes aware of his or her negative feelings and can begin exploring their root cause to find why these feelings exist, ultimately becoming more open to the message that perhaps eating meat is contributing to that negativity.

If you are to succeed in assisting others to overcome addictive and selfish behaviors, it will be due to compassionate communication, and if you succeed in pointing the way for others toward the liberating process of enlightenment, they will only be able to reach it through their own deep compassion. If you can convey this—if you can somehow graft compassion into the hearts of others by your example—you will have given them the greatest gift.

2. FEELING: The *Means* of Communication

If you want to truly communicate to others, then before you speak, ask yourself:

> How do I want them to feel about themselves when I talk to them?

One of the most inspiring speakers I know of is Dr. Martin Luther King, Jr. I have studied his speeches for years trying to glean a bit of what made him so effective, but it wasn't until I saw a documentary film about Malcolm X that I had an insight that gave me something new to consider regarding my own effectiveness as a speaker.

When Malcolm X spoke to African-Americans, he addressed them as victims. He took every opportunity to remind them how they had been victimized by whites. He did this, I think, in order to move them to action. He wanted them to be angry about the way they were being treated so that they would take justice into their own hands. He certainly had legitimate reasons to oppose the way blacks were being persecuted in America. However, I don't feel that he was effective in bringing about an enduring positive transformation because he perceived himself and his audience as victims.

Dr. King had a different approach. He did not see African-Americans as victims. He saw them as strong, whole, and complete. He didn't have time for hate, recognizing it as something that would slow him down on his way to his goal of racial equality. As he said, "I have decided to go with love. Hate is just too heavy a burden to bear." Dr. King envisioned a new world in which all people lived together in harmony, and he spoke from that elevated dream. Black people who heard him felt themselves to be strong, whole, and complete, empowered with vision and hope to take their rightful place in society rather than remain victims of an unjust racist system.

Only through humility and respect will you be effective in communicating. When conveying the messages of yoga and vegetarianism to others, it is important that you do not make them feel condemned or judged, but feel empowered to make conscious choices that would lead to liberation.

3. SEEING: The *Expression* of Communication

TO SEPARATE THE WORLD INTO GOOD GUYS AND BAD GUYS OR VICTIMS and perpetrators will only result in more division, not the peaceful unification we seek as yogis. When you engage in conversation with others who may not agree with your point of view, be sure that you are coming from a place of tolerance yourself. Dr. Martin Luther King, Jr., put it this way, "You have no moral grounding with someone who can feel your underlying contempt for them."

When you speak to others about vegetarianism or animal rights, you must not view them as stupid, callous, or evil. Instead, see them through your eyes of compassion. See them as holy beings, capable of kindness. If the person eats meat, why not view that as a temporary condition? If you can't see others as potentially kind and compassionate beings, how can you ever expect them to see themselves that way?

We must remember that all beings—including the animals—find themselves in their present situations due to past karmas. This is not to say that the animals deserve to be punished and that we should condone or even contribute to their suffering. On the contrary, it is vital and essential that we do everything possible to alleviate the suffering of others. Our own liberation from suffering depends upon it. To become spiritually activated is to feel the power of liberation operating within you. We must help the defenseless animal who is the victim of cruelty, and we must also extend our compassion to help liberate the human being who is the victim of his or her own blindness, which is the result of thousands of years of cultural conditioning. Only through compassion can real and lasting change take place.

When we accept that our karmas create our reality, we may awaken to a more compassionate understanding of the suffering of others. The law of karma is universal justice, designed not to punish, but rather to bring one to enlightened awareness through the empathetic understanding that arises through our past and present life experiences. An abused animal may have been a meat eater a wink of an eye ago. The hunter driving a pick-up truck sporting the bumper sticker "DEER ARE LIKE EGGS—THEY CAN BE POACHED" might reincarnate as the innocent lamb rescued by the Farm Sanctuary from the dead pile in back of a slaughterhouse. We just don't know. It's best, when interacting with anyone, to view all beings with compassion. The world certainly won't be any worse for it.

ч. BLISS: The *Result* of Successful Communication

ECSTASY IS THE TRUE GROUND OF BEING, AND IT PULSATES WITHIN YOU at all times. Recognize it and celebrate it in others, and you will find it in yourself. By not trying to tame, enslave, and exploit others, you allow them the right to pursue their true natures and, in doing so, you allow yourself the same adventure into bliss.

If we are to spiritually evolve and survive as a species, we must liberate ourselves from the lie that we are separate from the rest of life. The world is a reflection of ourselves. By living in harmony with the Earth, we can find our way back to our true Self. I am not suggesting that we go "back to nature." That is not possible because nature is with us now. It is who we are. Go within to experience the wildness of your own self: that living place of harmony, where true anarchy—Self-rule—is the rule.

Establish your goals. Recognize the potential within yourself to become liberated and for your life to serve as an instrument of liberation for others. Cultivate your vision through infusing yourself with vast compassion that extends to include everyone.

Never before in our known planetary history have we as individuals had such potential to decide our imminent future and that of this planet. If we are complacent and do nothing, the world as we know it will shut down. If, on the other hand, we come to our senses and dare to care about the suffering and happiness of others, we will abolish slavery in our lifetime and liberate ourselves in the process. Liberation, or *moksha,* is the goal of yoga, and ecstasy, or bliss, is its experience.

SPIRITUAL ACTIVATION

Angry thoughts disarray the heart
Pierce through the deformity with breath as your start
Shatter with a blow or a throw
You could do it inside a wishing well
Where your feelings once fell
If all else fails, embrace it with your holiness
Wrapping your everything around
Using the sound
Of the breath, what else could be better?
Yes that's it...the face of look upon you
Praying and Om-ing alone cannot do
Sitting at a lotus altar
While babies stumble to their slaughter

Nervous laughter holds you back from
Doing what you ought to
This Armageddon of look upon you
Is not going to stop, even in the forest, even in the shop
Hear the bodies going chop chop
It has only just begun
Birth is bloody—so many shades of red, she said
You don't know what it's like to be dead.
You heard them plotting to do disturbing things
What stopped you from intervening?
You are reeling in your obedience to ineffectualness.
Afraid of being humiliated? Stepping out of line?
Oh look at that face of look upon you!
Guilt paralyzes your mouth you cannot speak
Lies fill your ears, snuffing out the cries
Feet rooted in cement forgetfulness of who you are
So what to do?
Remember anyway and say something...anything
Pierce through the deformity
With a voice from the farm and the killing floor
When your own death is closing in
You will realize that the only thing
You ever really had in life was your effect upon others
Your end will come as a rattling snake slithering in
As you leave you will see that look upon you
You never ever had time, certainly no time to lose
Your body will stretch towards that last breath, so do your best
To see that all that you see is coming from inside of you
Nothing and no one has not been born from inside of you
Pierce through the deformity by means of breathing
Absorb into your rainbow body the pixilation of these phantoms
With the embrace of recognition
Allow black and white to collide into colors wondrous fair
And go on into the future of not knowing where.

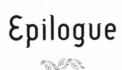

Epilogue

Blame keeps the sad game going. It keeps stealing all your wealth—giving it to an imbecile with no financial skills.
Dear one, wise up.
—HAFIZ

YOGA IS NOT FOR EVERYONE. YOGA IS FOR THOSE WHO WANT TO BE free and believe that *moksha* is possible. Not everyone wants to be free or even recognizes that they are in bondage. Not everyone realizes that through their own actions they could have an influence upon their own freedom and on the freedom of others. What others do is not ours to judge. Our work is the work on ourselves. We must embody what we feel is good and beautiful and not wait for others to lead us.

Anyone who comes to the practice of yoga at this time in the history of the world is not a beginner. To even have an interest in these ancient liberation practices is evidence of many lifetimes of previous practice. To be able to begin to comprehend the immensity that yoga offers, a person must already have some eligibility arising from past life experiences. A yogi is born with the desire to be free. Therefore yoga should not be proselytized. The missionary approach of converting the "ignorant savages" will not work when it comes to yoga. Trying to force people to "do" yoga because it is good for them or good for the planet is a ludicrous idea.

There are a growing number of yoga practitioners in the world today. We are incredibly privileged to be exposed to these ancient wisdom teachings and methods, which offer techniques for using compassion and kindness to bring about happiness and liberation. Human beings may have caused the present global crisis, but its disastrous consequences need not become a reality. The future of our planet can be determined by our actions now.

Liberation is not for everyone, but it may be for you. Yoga teaches the truth through direct experience, and the truth will set you free. Now the cage door is open, but no one will force us to walk out and leave our prison. The choice is ours alone. It is up to us and always has been. It is indeed possible for us to break the chains that bind us to the wheel of *samsara*. Whatever we want in life, we should first provide it for others. Through an understanding of how karma works, we come to realize the great impact of our own actions on the world. We realize that the bondage and suffering we experience in the world is caused by the bondage and suffering we inflict upon others. To liberate others is to liberate oneself.

Our relationship to animals is our relationship to nature. When we cease to enslave animals and cease to view them as exploitable, we break the chains of conditioning that have held us for thousands of years. When we say "no" to feeding upon the meat, milk, and blood of others, we say "yes" to liberation. We become liberated as spiritual beings, feeling a connection and sense of belonging to the living scheme of things.

Let go of judging others. Remember that they, like you, are only doing the best they can. When you point a blaming finger at someone else, keep in mind that there are three other fingers pointing back at you. By letting go of blaming others, you will find that you have a lot of time to devote to working on yourself. Don't try to change the whole world. Clean up your own house first. Eventually but inevitably you will come to see that as you become kinder, the world will become a kinder place.

Appendix I
Frequently Asked Questions

1. *Q: I just want to practice yoga for the physical benefits. Why should I be concerned with vegetarianism, the environment, or political activism?*

A: What could be more physical than what you eat, where you live, and whom you live with?

2. *Q: Human beings have always eaten meat. It's natural; even animals eat other animals. Shouldn't we as yogis try to live a more natural life?*

A: Some meat eaters defend meat eating by pointing out that it is natural; in the wild, animals eat one another. The animals that end up on our breakfast, lunch, and dinner plates, however, aren't those who normally eat other animals. The animals we exploit for food are not the lions and tigers and bears of the world. We eat the gentle vegan animals. However, on today's farms, we actually force them to become meat eaters by making them eat feed containing the rendered remains of other animals, which they would never eat in the wild.

Lions and other carnivorous animals do eat meat, but that doesn't mean we should. They would die if they didn't eat meat. Human beings, in contrast, choose to eat meat; it isn't a physiological necessity. In fact, we are designed anatomically to be vegetarians (see Question #4). Lions and other carnivorous animals do a lot of things besides eat meat. They live outdoors, not in houses; they don't wear clothes or drive around in cars. Why cite just one of the many things that they do and argue that we should imitate them? This doesn't make much sense.

Besides, there are many activities that human beings have been doing "forever." We might argue from that perspective that eating meat should be allowed to continue. Men have been raping women for thousands of years; does that mean that it is normal and should be allowed to continue? No, human beings came to recognize rape as a crime. Yogis investigate all long-standing habits and behaviors and evaluate them by one criterion: Does this activity bring me or the world closer to enlightenment?

It is wise for the yogi to consider that when someone causes harm to another that action perpetuates the wheel of *samsara*, the cycle of birth, life, and death. The yogi is attempting to be free of samsara and therefore does not eat meat since it creates the type of karma that keeps us bound to the wheel.

3. Q: What about Eskimos?

A: Everyone without exception must reap what they have sown. There is no escape from the law of karma. Because of the shortage of available vegetables, Arctic-dwelling Eskimos eat a large amount of meat and animal fat. They also have one of the highest incidences of heart disease and osteoporosis[40] in the world and, in general, short life spans.[41] That's something to consider.

4. Q: Aren't humans biologically designed to be meat eaters or at least omnivores?

A: The anatomical and physiological facts suggest no. We have small, flat mouths with small teeth. We don't have long, sharp canines to tear flesh. We have incisors in the front to bite and molars along the sides to chew and grind fruits and vegetables. Our teeth aren't strong enough to chew and crush hard things like raw bones, whereas carnivores can. We have a rotating jaw that moves from side to side, another useful feature for grinding plants. Carnivores and omnivores have hinge-joint jaws that open and close. They don't normally chew their food well before swallowing, and they don't need to. Unlike us, they don't have an abundance of the enzyme ptyalin in their saliva, which breaks down complex carbohydrates found only in plant foods. Once we have chewed and swallowed our food, it travels through a very long digestive tract, although not as long as that of our herbivore friends—the cows, horses, and sheep. Meat-eating species, comparatively, have short intestinal tracts, which allow them to move food through their systems quickly, so as not to allow rotting flesh to stagnate and cause disease.

Because we lack sharp claws, aren't very fast on our feet, and aren't exactly endowed with lightning reflexes, it would be very difficult if not impossible for us to run down an animal, catch it with our bare hands, and tear through its fur and skin in order to eat it. Biologically, we are designed to be frugivorous herbivores eating mainly fruits, seeds, roots, and leaves.

Humans do not need to eat the flesh of other animals to exist, whereas some animals are carnivores and cannot survive by eating only vegetables. Humans, on the other hand, eat meat only out of choice. We have been conditioned, taught, and coerced by the agents of our culture (parents, grandparents, advertisers, food critics, etc.) to eat the flesh and drink the milk of other animals. Because of this conditioning, which has occurred over a long period of time (thousands of years), we have

[40] R. Mazess, "Bone Mineral Content of North Alaskan Eskimos," Americal Journal of Clinical Nutrition 9 (1974): 916-925.

[41] Geoff Bond, Deadly Harvest: The Intimate Relationship Between Our Health and Our Food (Square One Publishers, 2007) 91.

developed addictive eating habits and blinded ourselves to the facts of our biological system and its true needs.

5. Q: If we all become vegetarians, will there be enough vegetables to feed all of us?

A: If we stop feeding grain to livestock, we will have enough food to feed all the starving human beings in the world. A reduction of meat consumption by only ten percent would yield enough grain to feed all the humans who starve to death each year worldwide—about sixty million.[42] Buddhist teacher Thich Nhat Hanh says: "Every day forty thousand children die in the world for lack of food. We who overeat in the West, who are feeding grains to animals to make meat, are eating the flesh of these children."[43]

6. Q: What would farm animals do if we stop eating them and let them go free? Where will they go? They've been domesticated for thousands of years; they don't know how to live on their own. Wouldn't it be a form of cruelty not to take care of them?

A: This is the same argument that white American slave owners gave in the 1800s when they tried to defend their right to own slaves. Yes, we have robbed these animals of their wildness, and they might not be able to revert to a feral state if all the doors of all the factory farms were opened. We have severely altered these animals biologically and emotionally, depriving them of any opportunity to develop skills with which to live with one another and their environment. This process of degradation has been going on for thousands of generations. The first step is to stop abusing these beings: stop breeding them through cruel, artificial means. It may be unrealistic to let them all go free right now, but it is realistic to acknowledge that, as a species, we human beings are quite ingenious. If we give serious consideration to this problem, we will no doubt find solutions and eventually free these animals. When we do, we will free ourselves.

7. Q: If yoga teaches us that all of life is sacred, then what is the difference if I eat a carrot or a hamburger?

A: Yes, all of life is sacred, and there is scientific evidence supporting the idea that plants have feelings. However, in the Yoga Sutras, Patanjali gives *ahimsa*, or nonharming, as a "practice," which implies that it can never be perfected. You practice doing your best to cause the *least* amount of harm. He also recommends *aparigraha*, which is the practice of not being greedy, or taking too much. The animals whom we eat consume large quantities of vegetables, so when you eat those animals you are consuming not only the animals but also all the vegetables that those animals have been eating.

---

[42] Boyce Resenberger, "Curb on US Waste Urged to Help World's Hungry," New York Times 25 Oct. 1974.
[43] Thich Nhat Hanh, Creating True Peace (New York: Simon & Schuster, 2003) 77.

Additionally, animals raised for human consumption require a lot of food and land. It takes eight or nine cows a year to feed one average meat eater. Each cow eats one acre of green plants, soybeans, and corn. So it takes nine acres of plants a year to feed one meat eater, compared with half an acre to feed one vegetarian.[44] Most of the plants grown to be fed to farm animals are heavily saturated with pesticides and herbicides and have been genetically modified, all of which contributes to the pollution and death of our environment. In terms of causing the least amount of harm, a vegetarian diet is superior, because a vegetarian eats the plants directly instead of eating the animals who were fed plants.

8. *Q: Isn't the real problem human overpopulation rather than meat eating?*

A: Human population growth is a problem in that most humans consume more than they need. The Earth's resources are now strained to sustain the needs and wants of the human population, which continues to escalate. The wealthier countries have curbed their population growth, in some cases to zero, while people in poorer or so-called "developing" countries give birth to many more babies on average. In the United States, the average is two children per family, while in Africa it is five children per family. On the surface, the statistic seems to indicate that Africans are having way too many kids and are taxing the Earth's resources, while American kids are born into families who are able to take care of them. However, the average American child consumes roughly the same resources as fifteen African children.[45] So when an American family says they only have two children, they are actually consuming the resources of an African family of thirty children! Furthermore, those American children will be indoctrinated into a lifestyle that teaches them to consume more than they need. Human overconsumption is a greater problem than human population growth, and meat eating is a big part of that problem. Some well-to-do parents may say, "I have a right to have as many children as I want because I can take care of them." That may be so, but can the Earth take care of them?

9. *Q: No one was so up in arms about meat eating until recently, with the rise of industrialized farming and the cruel practices common in today's factory farms. Couldn't we go back to a simpler way of raising animals for food and support only small family-owned farms where animals are treated humanely?*

A: Farms, whether small or large, are places where slaves are kept. The animals are fattened up to be eaten, or exploited for their ability to make honey or milk, or for their fur, wool or body parts; they are kept

---

[44] Marc Bekoff, Strolling With Our Kin (New York: Lantern Books, 2000) 70.

[45] Roger-Mark Desouza, Frederick Meyerson, and John S. Williams, "Critical Links: Population, Health and the Environment," Population Bulletin 58.3 (2003).

as breeders to produce more animals who can in turn be exploited and ultimately sold, slaughtered, and eaten. Some people may argue that if the animals are treated humanely prior to being slaughtered, this justifies their confinement and slaughter. Is it ethical to rob beings of their freedom but give them a comfortable prison and provide them with food until they become fat enough to be slaughtered? Any way you look at it, farms are places where animals are kept in preparation to be slaughtered and ultimately eaten as food. The question might be put this way: Is it really that much better to make friends with animals before you kill them than to treat them as nameless, faceless objects before you kill them? From a yogic point of view, one must weigh the karmic consequences of perceiving others as mere objects to be used and the consequences of profiting from the suffering of others.

10. *Q: Is there a difference between animal rights and animal welfare?*
A: Yes. Animal rights activists believe that animals exist for their own reasons, not to be used by human beings. Some animal rights activists take an abolitionist stance and feel that we have no moral right to exploit animals for any reason. Activist Ingrid Newkirk sums it up like this: Animals are not ours to eat, wear, experiment on, use for entertainment or for any exploitative purpose. Animal welfarists, on the other hand, do not believe that the lives of animals are important for their own sake. They believe that if we take care of animals and see to their welfare by providing them with a quality of life that gives them the appearance of happiness and health, it is okay to exploit them for our own purposes. Welfarists are concerned with the quality of the animals' lives before or even during their slaughter and want animals to be treated, and slaughtered, "humanely." Welfarists don't necessarily feel that it is wrong for humans to use animals for our own purposes.

11. *Q: Are animals a lower life form than humans?*
A: It has been an obsession of human beings to create a hierarchy that places the human species on top and lumps all the "other animals" together beneath us. The resulting "speciesism" allows us to look upon animals as less deserving of all manner of rights and considerations than humans. To support this lower status, humans have argued that animals act instinctually; don't have souls; don't feel physical pain like we do; and lack self-consciousness, cognitive intelligence, emotional feelings, morality, and ethics. In fact, numerous scientific laboratory tests and field observations have led to the conclusion that animals are conscious, intelligent, emotional beings. They are not machines and truly feel physical pain when it is inflicted upon them. They are capable of experiencing a

wide range of emotions, including loneliness, embarrassment, sadness, longing, depression, anxiety, panic, and fear, as well as joy, relief, surprise, happiness, contentment, and peace. At times some may exhibit behavior that shows a highly developed sense of morality and ethics. They may not speak human languages, although some primates have been taught American Sign Language (ASL); they nonetheless have highly developed communication skills and vocal languages of their own that no human being has yet mastered, except maybe Dr. Doolittle.

12. *Q: Why have human beings treated animals so poorly for so many years—enslaving, torturing, exploiting, and massacring them?*
A: That is the *big* question each of us must answer for the animals and ourselves. Perhaps we have treated them so poorly because we have the means to do so and can get away with it. Perhaps in a perverted attempt to feel powerful ourselves we exert power over others who are defenseless against our weapons of mass destruction (poisons, bombs, guns, spears, knives, forks, etc.). Perhaps, because of our unenlightenment, we do not know that what we do to others we ultimately do to ourselves. Perhaps because of our ignorance of who we really are, we strive for a sense of identity through dominating others. Perhaps we are so unconscious about our actions that we don't even realize the immense suffering we are causing to animals, the planet, and ourselves. Perhaps we have become so addicted to our greed-driven habits that we have lost our moral compass and don't know what is right and wrong. Perhaps we have just gone along with the crowd and haven't questioned our assumptions or our behavior in regard to our fellow earthlings. Perhaps common sense is not so common.

13. *Q: Are all meat eaters bad people, all vegans good people, and all animals innocent victims?*
A: No. Everyone is caught in the web of his or her own actions and is bound by past karmas (actions). *Good* and *bad* are relative terms. Every action takes one to the next place. One's knowledge of karma should not be used to judge others. You should ask yourself: Do I like where I am going, or do I want to change my direction? Through yoga practice you can change the course of your life by purifying your karma. But to do that you must have an idea of where you've been and where you want to go. Patanjali tells us that if we practice aparigraha, we will begin to understand not only where we have come from but where we are going and how our karmas have contributed to where we are now.

14. Q: What does it mean to be a spiritual person?
A: All living beings are spiritual beings because all of life breathes. Breath is an indication that spirit is present. The words for *spirit* in the ancient languages of Aramaic (*ruha*) and Hebrew (*ruach*) also mean "breath." Even in English, *breath* is defined as "the vital spirit, which animates living beings." Our breath is connected to the air that *every being* breathes. By breathing consciously, we acknowledge our communion with all of life. There are atoms of air in your lungs that were once in the lungs of everyone who has ever lived. In essence, we are breathing (inspiring) one another. To be alive is to be breathing. To live and breathe with an exclusive focus on one's small self, disconnected from the whole, is the definition of egotism. The enemy of the spirit is the selfish ego, which thinks that happiness can be gained through causing unhappiness and disharmony to others. In many ancient languages, the word for *enemy* means "one who falls out of rhythm; one who is not working in harmony with the larger group."[46]

Freedom from this disharmony can begin by letting go of the breath as "my" breath. As we let go, we enter into the shared life force, into a sense of harmony that connects us all: the breath, the Holy Spirit. If you want to know if someone is a "spiritual being" ask yourself, "Is he or she breathing?" If the answer is yes, then you know that you are in the presence of a spiritual being.

15. Q: Can you eat meat and still be a spiritual person?
A: All breathing beings are spiritual; this includes everyone who breathes, whether they are animals or humans, carnivores or vegetarians.

16. Q: Can someone be a meat-eating environmentalist?
A: If that someone is a human being, then in my opinion, no; it is a contradiction in terms. To be an environmentalist is to care about the environment and care about life on planet Earth. The raising of animals for food and all that it entails is the single most destructive force impacting our planet's fragile ecosystems. Our planet simply cannot sustain the greed of billions of human beings who are eating other animals.

17. Q: If the law of karma is true, then shouldn't we accept the fact that animals are suffering because of their karmas?
A: It is true that every being is enjoying life or suffering as a direct result of his or her own past actions. The animals in the factory farms may have been meat-eating human beings in a previous birth; we don't know, and it is not our place to judge. Nonetheless, their suffering provides us with an opportunity to step in and alleviate suffering where we see it. By choosing

---

[46] See Neil Douglas-Klotz, The Hidden Gospel: Decoding the Spiritual Message of the Aramaic Jesus (Wheaton, IL: Quest Books, 1999) 41–45.

to be kind instead of cruel, we can break the karmic chain of reacting to violence with more violence, contributing to a more peaceful future for everyone.

18. *Q: How can you care about animals when there is so much human suffering going on in the world?*
A: For compassion to truly be compassion, it can't discriminate. Compassion has to be limitless; it has to extend to all beings. If yogis are to come to the realization of the interconnectedness of life, then we must free ourselves from the conditioning that has caused us to think it is all right to exclude all the other animals from our own goals of peace, freedom, and happiness. We must stop viewing ourselves as separate and disconnected from the rest of life, as if we are a special case and the laws of nature do not apply to us. Besides, the way we treat animals is causing most of the human suffering in the world, from poverty, starvation, disease, and war to lack of clean air and water.

19. *Q: Shouldn't we as spiritual practitioners try to live a more simple life and just eat normal food and not be picky? Vegetarianism seems so complicated!*
A: It is a testament to the effectiveness of advertising campaigns funded by the animal-user industries that a diet that is bad for us and harmful to the planet is thought of as "normal" and a diet that promotes health, happiness, and well-being is thought of as alternative, abnormal, or faddish. In fact, these days it is relatively easy to find vegetarian options in many restaurants and supermarkets, though you may have to ask. Moreover, the fact is that it is much more complicated to confine, raise, feed, slaughter, process, package, and market an animal for food than it is to grow plants.

20. *Q: I don't eat meat, but I eat fish. Isn't that all right? Isn't it true that fish are cold-blooded and don't feel pain?*
A: Actually, fish are very sensitive creatures with highly developed nervous systems. They feel pain acutely. If they weren't able to feel pain, they, like us, could not have survived as a species. Their nervous systems, like ours, secrete opiate-like pain-dampening biochemicals in response to pain.[47] Here is an example that may help you understand just how sensitive a fish is. If you were a fish, and you were to touch a doorknob, you would be able to *feel* the presence of every person who had touched that doorknob during the course of a day.[48] Have you seen how fish are able to swim in a school so precisely relating to their fish-fellows and never clumsily bump into one another? That's because they have a highly developed sense of feeling in their bodies, which enables them to feel not

---

[47] Pamela Rice, 10 Reasons Why I'm a Vegetarian (New York: Lantern Books, 2005) 168-169.
[48] Peter Redgrove, The Black Goddess and the Unseen Real (New York: Grove Press, 1987) 21.

only the movement of the water against their skin but the presence of other beings who are close.

Fishing is not a benign activity; it is hunting in the water. Fish are complex beings who choose mates, use words to communicate, build nests, cooperate with one another to find food, have long-term memories, and use tools.

Visit: www.nofishing.net or www.pisces.demon.co.uk.

21. Q: At least if we choose to eat fish, it's cleaner for the environment and we aren't contributing to the ecological toll that eating beef or pork is causing, right?

A: Wrong. Fishing is taking a huge toll on the planet's ecosystem. We are emptying the oceans, seas, lakes, and rivers as we fish them dry. Large factory trawlers indiscriminately scrape and haul up everything from the ocean floor, along with everyone unfortunate enough to get caught in the nets. Roughly one-third of what is dragged in is not profitable fish, but other sea animals, including turtles, whales, dolphins, seals, and sea birds.[49] These beings are referred to by the fishing industry as "by-catch." Severely traumatized and wounded, these animals are subsequently thrown back into the ocean, dead or dying.

To meet the huge consumer demand for fish, the industry can no longer rely on hunting wild fish. Now we are doing to fish what was done to wild cows, sheep, goats, chickens, and ducks thousands of years ago: we are confining them in holding pens. These floating fish farms or hatcheries, like their land equivalents, are sites for genetic engineering. They contribute to polluting the ocean with toxic excrement and residue as any other farm would. Many genetically "altered" fish escape from the confines of the crowded floating concentration camps to mingle and mate with their wild fish cousins, causing horrible and irreversible damage to wild species.

Today's fishing industry supplies land farms with fish as well. Over fifty percent of the fish caught is fed to livestock on factory farms and "regular" farms.[50] It is an ingredient in the enriched "feed meal" fed to livestock. Farm animals, like cows, who by nature are vegans, are routinely force-fed fish as well as the flesh, blood, and manure of other animals. It may take sixteen pounds of grain to make one pound of beef, but it also takes one hundred pounds of fish to make that one pound of beef.[51]

22. Q: Is it okay to drink organic milk?

A: Cows that are fed organic food are still kept as slaves on farms, regardless of whether it is a large corporate factory farm or a small family farm. As a yoga practitioner with some understanding of how karma works,

---

[49] Tuttle, The World Peace Diet, 102.
[50] S. Holt, "The Food Resources of the Ocean," Scientific American 221 (1969): 178-194.
[51] Watson, "Consider the Fishes," VegNews, 27.

you have to ask the question, "If I am seeking liberation, will it serve my purpose to rob other beings of their freedom?" We ourselves can never be free if we rob others of their freedom. Besides, every dairy cow, no matter what she has been fed, ends up in the slaughterhouse.

23. *Q: Don't cows need to be milked? Isn't it cruel not to milk them?*
A: A cow, like other mammals (including human females), doesn't give milk unless she is pregnant or has given birth to a baby. The milk her body produces is intended to provide nourishment for her baby. In our modern dairies, calves never get to nurse from their mothers longer than a few hours. They are taken away and fed synthetic formulas laden with growth-stimulating drugs and other pharmaceuticals, while we steal the milk for ourselves. Farmers profit financially from this theft and degradation. We are the only animals who steal and drink the milk from other species.

Dr. Benjamin Spock, a leading authority on child nutrition, printed an apology in the eighth edition of his best-selling book *Baby and Child Care* for ever suggesting feeding cow's milk to babies. He also advised a vegetarian diet for children, writing that children can get plenty of protein and iron from vegetables, beans, and other plant foods and thus avoid the fat and cholesterol in animal products.

24. *Q: Aren't cows sacred to yogis? Aren't milk and ghee considered perfect* sattvic *foods for a yogi?*
A: Yoga may have originated in India, where the cow has been revered as sacred for thousands of years, but times have changed since Lord Krishna played his flute for the cows of Vrindavan. There are factory farms in India now. European cows have been inbred with the native cows of India, resulting in a short-legged breed that is no longer useful in the heavy work of pulling carts or plowing fields. This doesn't limit the ability of the cows to produce milk, but approximately half the calves born are male. What happens to all the male calves being born in dairies? Their bodies wind up in the large black market focusing on beef and the sale of other products derived from cows. India is the leading exporter of leather to America and Europe. The tanning process involved in the leather is highly toxic and maims or kills thousands of people every year. Since it is illegal in many Indian states to kill a cow, there is much denial and secrecy surrounding the exploitation of cows in India.

25. *Q: How can I get enough protein if I eat a vegan diet?*
A: The required daily amount (RDA) of protein is fifty to seventy grams, which is easily met by eating a wide assortment of plant foods. It is a myth

that only animal products contain protein. There is protein in beans and grains as well as in almonds, broccoli, mushrooms, avocados, and even potatoes. There is another myth, which says that you must carefully combine proteins from plant sources in each meal to meet the RDA. This is not true. Simply eat a variety of different plant foods over the course of a day, and you will meet your protein requirements. Read the book *Hope's Edge* by Frances and Anna Moore Lappe for more information.

26. Q: Can I get vitamin B12 on a vegan diet?

A: A vegan must rely on getting adequate vitamin B12 from a supplement or from eating foods that have been fortified with vitamin B12. If we weren't so dirt-conscious, we would obtain adequate vitamin B12 from soil, air, water, and bacteria, but we meticulously wash and peel our vegetables now—and with good reason, as we can't be sure our soil is not contaminated with pesticides and herbicides. Today "aged" foods like sauerkraut, miso, and tempeh are fermented in hygienically sanitized stainless-steel vats to assure cleanliness, so we can no longer be sure they will provide us with the B12 we need. Vegans should not mess around with this issue. To ensure that you are getting the tiny amount (2.5 micrograms) you need per day, take a supplement and/or drink fortified soymilk or rice milk. Read the book *Becoming Vegan* by Brenda Davis, R.D., and Vesanto Melina, M.S., R.D., for more information.

27. Q: Don't I need to drink milk to get enough calcium?

A: No. In fact, drinking milk and eating dairy products can rob your body of calcium and contribute to osteoporosis. If you eat dark green leafy vegetables like kale, collards, and mustard greens, you can get enough calcium from a vegan diet. Beans, tofu, cabbage, and broccoli are additional sources of calcium. If you doubt that you are meeting the thousand milligram RDA, include calcium-fortified foods like fruit juice, cereals, soy or grain beverages, or take a supplement. Also, the weight-bearing aspect of yoga asana practice contributes to bone density and health. Sunlight is essential to the body's ability to absorb calcium from the food you are eating. Make sure you receive adequate vitamin D every day through sunlight. About fifteen to twenty minutes of sun on the face and hands is usually enough for most of us. Read the book *CalciYum* by David and Rachel Bronfman for more information and recipes.

28. Q: How do I become a vegan?

A: You could begin gradually by, for example, being vegan one day a week. Choose a day, and on that day don't eat any meat, milk, eggs, or fish. This would make a big difference to your health and to the environment. Alternatively, you can try giving up meat and dairy foods one at a time, quitting milk, fish, eggs, or meat, etc. Remember that you are not inflicting punishment upon or depriving yourself, but rather fostering a longer, happier, healthier life for you and the planet. Or just immediately stop participating in the cruelty; just stop, period. Why, if you know the truth about how animals are treated, would you want to eat them ever again? The truth shall set you free. The door of your cage is open, just walk out. Why not go for it? Be totally free. Leave the cage forever and never go back.

29. *Q: How can I be an effective speaker and use my words to move people to be more compassionate toward animals and stop eating them?*

A: Be a joyful vegan yourself. View everyone as providing you with opportunities to be kind and to articulate empathy and compassion for another being. See whomever you speak to as a holy being. Do not see anyone as mean, stupid, compassionless, or as a person who needs you to enlighten him or her. If you can't see people you speak to as compassionate, how can you ever expect them to see themselves that way?

Before you speak to someone, ask yourself: How do I want this person to feel about him- or herself? Do you have the largeness of heart to see that person's highest potential? For that to occur, you must be willing to give up any negative thoughts about him or her in order to provide a space for the person to turn around in. Keep in mind that when you are speaking to others, they can always *feel* your underlying contempt or respect for them, and that will determine whether they are able to hear your message. What is your goal in speaking to them? Is it to vent your anger, to assert your superiority, to berate them, or to make them feel guilty? Or do you really want to empower them to change for the better and to become the kind of people who don't cause animals to suffer? If you really want them to stop eating meat, you must see in them the potential to do that, and you must speak to that potential.

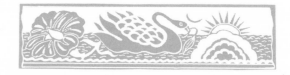

Appendix 2
Getting Started on a Vegan Diet

21 Day Cleansing Diet

MANY DOCTORS AGREE THAT IT TAKES ABOUT THREE WEEKS (TWENTY-ONE DAYS) for the human digestive system to rid itself of toxins and to free us from destructive eating habits and biochemical addictions. Meat and dairy eating is addictive. How is this possible? Dr. Neal Barnard explains in his book *Breaking the Food Seduction*: "Scientific tests suggest that meat may have subtle drug-like qualities…. As meat touches your tongue opiates are released in the brain…. Meat stimulates a surprisingly strong release of insulin…. In turn, insulin is involved in the release of dopamine between brain cells. Dopamine…is the ultimate feel-good chemical turned on by every single drug of abuse—opiates, nicotine, cocaine, alcohol, amphetamines, and everything else."[52] Dr. Barnard makes a similar point about cheese.

First, viewing yourself with compassion is essential for the success of any diet program. Guilt-tripping and negative projection are never helpful. If you can free yourself from your destructive addictions, you will discover that within your own body is a pharmaceutical laboratory that can provide you with the well-being you seek. But to become independent you must first give yourself the chance of experiencing your body when it is not hampered by addiction, so you can begin to feel its innate intelligence.

You may feel that going from the Standard American Diet (SAD) of meat and dairy products to a one hundred percent organic vegan diet overnight may be too much. Or maybe your schedule is too busy to allow you to stay on it for the full twenty-one days. The important thing is not to beat yourself up and feel pressured to change overnight. Instead, just try this diet for one day without feeling you have to commit to a vegan diet for the whole rest of your life. Even one day will be greatly appreciated by your body and mind and by the animals as well as the greater world we all share.

But if you are up for the full adventure, then following this simple diet for twenty-one days will give your digestive organs a rest and will gently help them to transition to a healthier diet. This diet will reset your metabolism and help free you from biochemical addictions triggered by food, drugs, and emotions.

---

[52] Neal Barnard, M.D, <u>Breaking the Food Seduction</u> (New York: St. Martin's Griffin, 2003) 63-64.

This is by no means a starvation diet; it provides ample food and lots of fiber. You will find that you are not hungry, nor will you have problems with constipation. This diet is vegan, eliminating all animal-based foods. In addition, it also eliminates wheat and soy, because sometimes these foods cause allergic reactions. Oil is eliminated as well, to help you lose unwanted weight and to give the gall bladder and liver a rest from the job of metabolizing fat. Drugs, alcohol, and caffeine are eliminated to help clear the thinking mind and allow you to reflect on how you deal with stress. The elimination of drugs, alcohol, and caffeine also provides the nervous system and internal organs—especially the liver and kidneys—a rest from having to process these challenging substances.

Salt and sugar are taken in minimal amounts. You will get some salt from the seaweed in the nightly kitchari soup, and you will get some natural sugar in the fruit and juice. Eliminating salt will help release fluids from your tissues and reduce swelling and puffiness. Many times when we feel we look "fat," it is not fat we are seeing but water retention. Eliminating sugar helps the overall metabolism to become more balanced, stable, and less prone to cravings and binges.

As the food that you will eat will be blended or porridge-like, it will aid in digestion and give your jaw a rest.

Make sure that all you do choose to eat is organic so as to minimize adding any new toxins to your own bodily system or into the greater system we all share: the Earth.

You will eat two meals a day—oatmeal for breakfast and a porridge-like soup and blended salad for dinner—with a lunch snack.

Here is a list of the staple food items you will need to have on hand:

Old-fashioned oatmeal (not instant or prepackaged)
Oat bran
Brown rice
Red lentils
Split green peas
Kombu seaweed
Apples
Carrots
Beets
Lemons
Cucumbers
Tomatoes

Leafy dark greens: a fresh assortment
(lettuce, parsley, arugula, kale, dandelion, etc.)
Raw sauerkraut
Powdered spirulina (blue-green algae)
An assortment of herbal non-caffeinated teas
Laxative tea

Supplements—try to get all organic and vegan (no gelatin capsules):
Aloe vera juice (preferably with pulp)
Digestive enzymes
Acidophilus (nondairy) in tablets or capsules
Silica (horsetail) (helps to promote strong and shiny
hair and glowing skin)
Multivitamins
Vitamin B12

The following appliances will make your meal preparation easier:
Blender or food processor
Large soup pot
(stainless steel—not aluminum or Teflon-coated)
Small saucepan
(stainless steel—not aluminum or Teflon coated)

The Diet Plan

Breakfast
Upon rising:
• Take digestive enzymes and acidophilus on an empty stomach and drink
1-2 oz. of aloe vera juice.
• Drink a cup of herbal tea without any milk or sweeteners—chamomile,
peppermint, and licorice are good options.

After 20 minutes:
• Eat a bowl of plain oatmeal without adding salt, sugar, soymilk, or any
other kind of milk. After eating the oatmeal, take the multivitamin, B12,
and silica tablets.

Lunch Snack
• If you feel hungry during the day, drink more herbal tea or some fresh vegetable or fruit juice (not bottled, canned, or processed) and lots of water.

Dinner
• 20 minutes before eating, drink an 8 oz. glass of room temperature water, take digestive enzymes and acidophilus, and drink 1-2 oz. of aloe vera juice.
• Eat a bowl of kitchari.
• Eat a bowl of blended raw salad.
• Eat at least 2 tablespoons of raw sauerkraut.

How to make oatmeal
Place ½ cup raw oats in a saucepan, and add 2 cups of cold water. Bring to a boil, reduce heat to low, simmer for 10 minutes, and serve. This makes a very creamy, soup-like porridge.

How to make kitchari
Measure out 1½ cups dry red lentils (or split green peas) and ½ cup brown rice. Place in large soup pot and add 10 cups of water and a 4-inch piece of dry kombu seaweed. The seaweed affects the chemistry of the lentils (as well as other beans), rendering them more digestible. Bring to a boil and then simmer for about 1 hour. If you make a big batch, you can refrigerate it and use it over a few days. Just reheat and add water if necessary.

How to make blended salad
Place all the ingredients that you might normally put in a large salad in a blender or food processor. Add 1 tablespoon lemon juice, 1 cup of cold water, and blend. (Do not add any oil, vinegar, salt, or pepper!)

Here are some suggested ingredients for your blended salad:

> 1/2 apple
> 1/2 carrot
> 1/2 beet
> 1/2 cucumber

3 cherry tomatoes
6 romaine lettuce leaves
6 arugula leaves
1 teaspoon spirulina (blue-green algae) powder

Make your own sauerkraut

It's actually easy. Check out **www.wildfermentation.com** for a recipe or buy some, but make sure it's raw.

Every night for the first week, drink a cup of herbal laxative tea before bedtime to get the elimination process going, then taper off and only drink it if you are having trouble eliminating in the morning.

Appendix 3
Yoga on the Mat

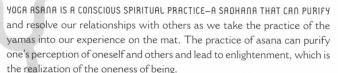

YOGA ASANA IS A CONSCIOUS SPIRITUAL PRACTICE—A SADHANA THAT CAN PURIFY and resolve our relationships with others as we take the practice of the yamas into our experience on the mat. The practice of asana can purify one's perception of oneself and others and lead to enlightenment, which is the realization of the oneness of being.

Enlightened yogis know that they are not the body nor the mind, but rather, that they "have" bodies and minds. The true Self is eternal. It can be challenging to realize that, however. Our bodies are made of our past karmas, which propel us into the experience of birth, which, in turn, is our opportunity to live and to realize who we really are beyond the vehicle that is the body/mind container.

Asana means "seat," and *seat* means connection to the Earth. Earth implies all beings and things. *Chakra* means "wheel." A chakra is a doorway through which we perceive reality. Our ability to see into the various dimensions of reality is reflected in the energetic ease or dis-ease found in our relationships. The disease of feeling disconnected from oneself and others is pervasive in our time. This disconnection causes us to hurt and exploit others, which only results in unhappiness and disease for others as well as ourselves.

Each asana corresponds to a specific chakra, as well as to a specific relationship. The practice of asana is a practical method for purifying our relationships, ultimately revealing to us our true nature as not separate, but as interconnected with all beings.

Karma means "action" and includes every thought, word, and deed we have done. The fact is, we do not act alone—our thoughts, words, and deeds are done in relation to others. Our karmas bind us to our relationships with others. Because our bodies are made of our past karmas, every asana provides an opportunity to access and heal these relationships. The purification of our relationships brings about a healing of the disease of disconnection and the reestablishment of a sound body and sound mind, able to embody, radiate, and communicate peace and joy to all.

If you preface your asana practice with the intention to resolve past relationships, then, while you are in each asana, allow the experience to help you remember those past relationships. If pain, doubt, or tightness arise, give silent blessings to the others in your life. The following descriptions might help you to reflect on the power of asana practice to heal relationships by resolving them into love, forgiveness, and blessing while on the mat.

1st Chakra: MULADHARA
(Root Place)
Standing Poses

Karmic relationships:
Mother Earth, nature, parents, home, job, money, boss, workplace

Your spiritual journey begins with acknowledging your physicality through devotion to the Great Goddess, Mother Nature. If you cannot be at peace with your parents and feel contentment with your body, home, and job, you won't be able to evolve. You purify the foundation by seeing all of life as sacred. Your connection to the Earth must be based in steadiness and joy, not only for yourself, but also for the whole world and all beings.

 The practice of standing poses develops stability and removes fear.

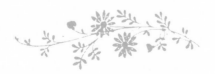

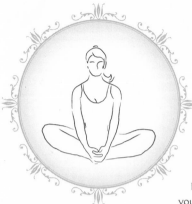

2nd Chakra: SWADHISHTHANA
(Her Favorite Standing Place)
Forward Bends

Karmic relationships:
Creative, artistic, romantic, and
sexual partners

You can purify your creative/sexual relationships by letting go of anger, blame, and resentment. Through practice, you will come to realize that the way others treat you is coming from how you have treated others in your past. Forward bending takes you into your past with an opportunity to reflect and heal through letting go of resentful feelings you may be holding against past partners.

 The practice of forward bending develops creativity and removes sorrow and envy.

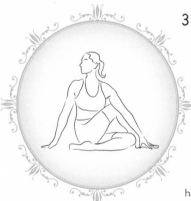

3rd Chakra: MANIPURA
(Jewel in the City)
Twists

Karmic relationships:
Others you have hurt (especially
focus on animals you may have
eaten or caused to be harmed)

Twisting asanas provide a great opportunity to reflect upon the food you have eaten and the other animal beings you may have harmed in the process. Acknowledge your unwitting selfishness and ask for forgiveness. Don't feel guilty. What you have already done in your past is done; you cannot change that, but you can move forward in a new and more compassionate way, starting now. Realize that when you hurt others, it is coming from a lack of self-confidence. This practice provides the means to remedy that.

 The practice of twists develops confidence and removes anger.

4th Chakra: ANAHATA
(Unstruck)
Backbends

Karmic relationships: Others who have hurt you

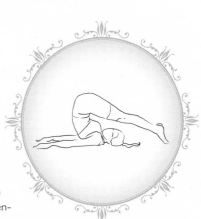

Have the largeness of heart to let go, forgive others, and move on. Know that others, just like you, are only doing the best they can in any given situation. Backbends allow you to move into the future. The ease that you have in moving into your future will be reflected in the ease you have with forgiving others.

 The practice of backbending develops compassion and forgiveness and removes hate and hostility.

5th Chakra: VISHUDDHA
(Poison Removing)
Shoulderstand, Plough, Fish

Karmic relationship: Yourself

Purification of this chakra helps you to develop *satya*, purity of speech, allowing you to say what you mean and to mean what you say. It enables you to see yourself as a holy being able to uplift the lives of others. If you are to attain enlightenment, you must begin to see yourself as deserving. When you vow to attain enlightenment so that you may contribute to the happiness and liberation of others, you will be freed of arrogance and cynicism in connection to your own self-image.

 The practice of shoulderstand develops the ability to communicate and removes cynicism.

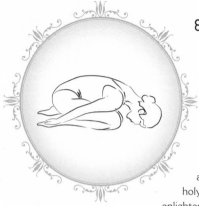

6th Chakra: AJNA
(Command Center)
Child's Pose

Karmic relationship: Teachers

When you bow to another as your teacher, the potent elixir of humility purifies you, releasing you from selfishness, jealousy and pride. You are then no longer attached to ego. A truly holy being is a humble being. *Guru* means "the enlightenment principle," and it operates through your teachers. When you see your teachers as holy, you tap into the power that can uplift the world!

 The practice of child's pose develops humility and removes doubt.

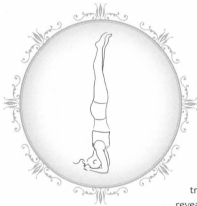

7th Chakra: SAHASRARA
(Thousand-Petaled Lotus)
Headstand

Karmic relationship: The Divine or Higher Self

What is realized in the yogic state of *samadhi* is the oneness of being, the sacred unity of all. Separateness is transcended as the light of cosmic awareness reveals the unity between the individual, nature, and the Divine.

 The practice of headstand can lead to the development of enlightenment and remove disconnection.

Resources

Books

* *101 Reasons Why I'm a Vegetarian* by Pamela Rice
* *Animals as Persons* by Gary Francione
* *Animal Liberation* by Peter Singer
* *An Unnatural Order* by Jim Mason
* *Battered Birds; Crated Herds* by Gene Bauston
* *Becoming Vegan* by Brenda Davis, R.D., and Vesanto Melina, M.S., R.D.
* *Breaking the Food Seduction* by Neal Barnard, M.D.
* *Diet for a New America* by John Robbins
* *Dominion* by Matthew Scully
* *Empty Cages* by Tom Regan
* *Eternal Treblinka* by Charles Patterson
* *Farm Sanctuary* by Gene Baur
* *Green Yoga* by George and Brenda Feuerstein
* *Gods of Love and Ecstasy* by Alain Danielou
* *Hope's Edge* by Frances and Anna Moore Lappe
* *Making Kind Choices* by Ingrid Newkirk
* *One Can Make a Difference* by Ingrid Newkirk
* *Peace to All Beings* by Judy Carman
* *Seeds of Deception* by Jeffrey M. Smith
* *Skinny Bitch* by Rory Freedman and Kim Barnouin
* *Slaughterhouse* by Gail Eisnitz
* *Strolling with Our Kin* by Marc Bekoff
* *Thanking the Monkey* by Karen Dawn
* *The China Study* by T. Colin Campbell, Ph.D., and Thomas M. Campbell II
* *The Food Revolution* by John Robbins
* *The Inner Art of Vegetarianism* by Carol J. Adams

* *The Mad Cowboy* by Howard Lyman
* *The Textbook of Yoga Psychology* by Shri Brahmananda Sarasvati
* *The World Peace Diet* by Will Tuttle, Ph.D.
* *Your Right to Know* by Andrew Kimbrell

Films

* *Chew on This*
* *Cow*
* *Earthlings*
* *I Am an Animal*
* *Meet Your Meat*
* *Peaceable Kingdom*
* *The Animals Film*
* *The Witness*

Organizations

* Abolitionist Approach: www.abolitionistapproach.com
* Animal Mukti: www.animalmukti.org
* Farm Sanctuary: www.farmsanctuary.org
* Howard Lyman Factoids & Links: www.madcowboy.com
* Humane Society of the United States: www.hsus.org
* Jivamukti Yoga: www.jivamuktiyoga.com
* Karen Dawn Media reports: www.DawnWatch.com
* PETA: www.peta.org
* Physicians Committee for Responsible Medicine: www.PCRM.org
* Vegan Outreach: www.veganoutreach.org

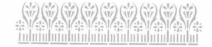

Glossary

abhinivesha: excessive fear of death, one of the five *kleshas*, or obstacles to Self-realization

abhyasa: *as* (to throw) + *abhi* (toward); to throw oneself into something; steady continuous practice; repeated endeavor. Abhyasa leads to spiritual development and wisdom.

abolitionist: someone who wants to abolish, or do away with, slavery

ahimsa: *a* (not) + *himsa* (harming); the practice of nonharming or nonviolence

antu: may it be so

aparigraha: greedlessness

asana: seat; the practice of connecting well to the Earth and all beings

asmita: identification with ego or personality self; one of the five kleshas, or obstacles to Self-realization

asteya: nonstealing

avidya: ignorance; mistaking oneself, others, or reality for what it is not; perceiving reality as existing as other or separate from oneself; unenlightened thinking that you are an individual who exists disconnected from the whole—not holy; one of the five kleshas, or obstacles to Self-realization

bhav: the Divine mood of unity; feeling holy—connected to the whole

brahmacharya: *brahma* (Hindu god of creativity or the creative power of becoming) + *charya* (vehicle or a means to move or reach toward); continence or the ability to specifically direct sexual energy toward spiritual awakening; not using sex selfishly to manipulate others

dharana: concentration; the practice of taking the mind from a fragmented disconnected state to a place of focus and wholeness; the necessary prerequisite to meditation

dharma: to support; fix in place; that which holds together

genetically modified organisms (GMO): organisms with genes that have been manipulated and altered. Human beings are genetically modifying both plants and animals, causing mutations to occur in the name of profit. No real benefit to human health or to animals, plants, or the ecosystem has resulted from this practice.

hatha yoga: uniting or joining the sun and the moon who represent self and other

himsic: harmful

Holy Scriptures: channeled words of wisdom intended to provide inspiration and guidance to spiritual aspirants, written by rishis and sages; some examples would be: The Bible, Koran, Vedas, Upanishads, Yoga Sutras, Hatha Yoga Pradipika, and the Bhagavad Gita

kirtan: praise; singing the names of God in a call-and-response manner. Kirtan as a practice "cuts" through the thinking mind.

klesha: hindrance; obstacle. Patanjali lists five kleshas or hinderances to the attainment of Yoga: *avidya* (ignorance), *asmita* (egoism), *raga* (attachment to what you like), *dvesha* (aversion to what you don't like), and *abhinivesha* (fear of death).

lokah: location

jiva: individual soul

jivanmukta: a liberated soul

jivanmukti: the state of liberation

memes (pronounced meems): the blueprints of a civilization, culture, or way of living that become implanted in the minds of each member of that culture and remain there unquestioned, becoming "mainstream" ideology

moksha: liberation

mukti: liberation; freedom from avidya

pranayama: to control the life force in order to expand or set it free; the fourth of the eight-limbed Ashtanga method of Yoga as outlined by Patanjali

pratishthayam: to be well-established or grounded in a certain practice; the result of abhyasa

Raja yoga: yoga for the king; the yoga system outlined by the eight limbs of Ashtanga yoga [*ashta* (eight) + *anga* (limb or attachment)]

satsang: *sat* (truth) + *anga* (limb or attachment); association with and attachment to the truth tantra: *tan* (to stretch) + *tra* (to cross over); various techniques or methods used to stretch or expand consciousness, enabling one to cross over avidya

sadhana: conscious spiritual practice

samadhi: *sam* (same) + *adhi* (highest); enlightenment; ecstasy; perfect absorption; Yoga

samsara: *sam* (same) + *sara* (agitation); to be repeatedly agitated; the cycle of rebirth

satya: truthfulness

sattvic: pure; balanced; clear

shunyata: emptiness; void; lacking qualities of its own. It is equated with the feminine principle, referring to that which is vast and boundless in its potential. Reality is empty and appears according to how the seer sees it. How the seer sees it is dependent upon his or her own karmas.

siddhi: power or extraordinary skill that arises through the practice of yoga

sukha: good space; centered in happiness; joy; freedom from suffering

vinyasa: *vi* (ordered placement) + *nyasa* (to place on purpose in a special way in a sequence); acting consciously or mindfully in each moment of time so that the sequence of actions leads to the desired outcome; a way of practicing yoga asanas in which a sequential, ordered placement is linked with conscious breath and intention designed to bring about *nirodha*, the cessation of the fluctuations of the mind

viveka: discriminating wisdom; the ability to know what is real, true, or eternal and what is unreal, false, or impermanent

yama: restriction

Yoga: the state of enlightenment; samadhi; ecstasy; the realization of the oneness of being and the dissolving of separateness

yoga: the practices done in order to attain enlightenment or to realize the oneness of being

Acknowledgements

To Victor Schonfeld and Myriam Alaux, the makers of the documentary that changed my life and put me on the path of animal activism and veganism, *The Animals Film*, and to Robert Wyatt, who composed the film's soundtrack. To Raoul Goff, Lisa Fitzpatrick, Arjuna van der Kooij, Brenda Knight, Mary Teruel, and Lucy Kee of Mandala Publishing for the courage to continuously strive to provide us with books that truly enrich our lives, and for giving me the opportunity to write this one. Huge appreciation goes to my dear friend and long-time editor Debra DeSalvo for helping me to actualize the book. Without her phenomenal editing assistance, this book would not have come to completion. My appreciation also goes to Vallabhdas, Paul Steinberg, Lois Laxmi Hill, Jaimie Epstein, and Banka, for stepping in at the last minute not only to help me straighten out my footnote issues but also to proof the text and provide meticulous copy edits. To David Life for reading the early manuscript and providing valuable insights, as well as continuous emotional and technical support. To my holy teachers, Shri Brahmananda Sarasvati, Swami Nirmalananda, Sri K. Pattabhi Jois, and Shyamdas, who have taught me the value of Sanskrit and continue to teach me the meaning and value of compassion. I am in awe and am continuously grateful to the growing number of Jivamukti Yoga teachers who have embraced animal rights and find clever as well as courageous ways to bring the message of veganism into the classes they teach. To my dear friends and fellow activists who inspire me to continue to be radical and speak up for the animals, even when faced with ridicule, attack, and violent opposition: Ingrid Newkirk, Michael Franti, Julia Butterfly Hill, Russell Simmons, John Robbins, Gene Baur, Martin Rowe, Will Tuttle,

Jim Mason, Jannette Patterson, Karen Dawn, Matthew Scully, Howard Lyman, Janet Rienstra, Kathy Freston, Kathy Stevens, and Jenny Brown. I want to acknowledge the work of Jim Mason, who wrote *An Unnatural Order*, and Will Tuttle, author of *The World Peace Diet*. If you found my book to be helpful, I encourage you to read their books, as they go deeper into the historical aspects of our culture's attitude toward animals and nature. Most importantly I wish to acknowledge all the animals whom I have hurt in my past. I apologize for my ignorance and the ignorance of my species and hope that with this book we can begin to heal the many wounds we have inflicted upon all of you: members of the animal nations, our fellow earthlings with whom we share life on this planet.

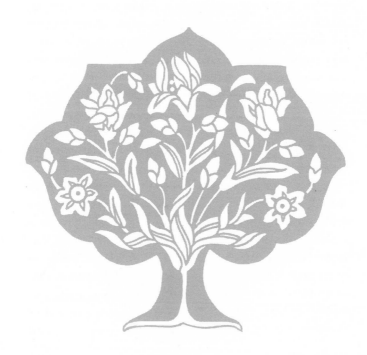

Colophon

The main text was typeset in Cantoria.
The main header text was typeset using TableManners.

Text printed on 60# Nature's Book Smooth Antique Recycled Paper.

Publisher & Creative Director
Raoul Goff

Art Director
Iain R. Morris

Managing Editor
Jake Gerli

Editors
Arjuna van der Kooij
Lucy Kee

Production Manager
Leslie Cohen

Designer
Mary Teruel

Figure Illustrations
Lallo Lemos

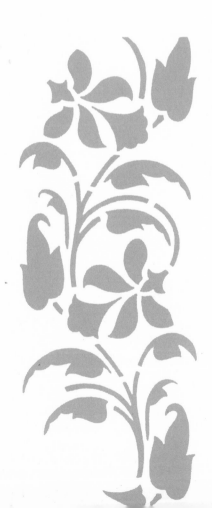